Xuē J

正體類要

Categorized Essentials of Repairing the Body

Zhèng Tǐ Lèi Yào

Lorraine Wilcox, L.Ac.

The Chinese Medicine Database
www.cm-db.com
Portland, Oregon

Categorized Essentials of Repairing the Body

正體類要

Zhèng Tǐ Lèi Yào

Lorraine Wilcox

Copyright © 2017 The Chinese Medicine Database

1017 SW Morrison #307A
Portland, OR 97205 USA

COMP designation original Chinese work and English translation

Cover Design by Jonathan Schell L.Ac.
Library of Congress Cataloging-in-Publication Data:

Xuē Jǐ, fl. 1487 - 1559
    [Categorized Essentials of Repairing the Body. English]
    Zheng Ti Lei Yao = Categorized Essentials of Repairing the Body.
    / translation Lorraine Wilcox
           p. cm.
    Includes Index.
    ISBN 978-0-9906029-3-4 (alk. paper)
    Medicine, Chinese   I. Wilcox, Lorraine. II. Title: Categorized
    Essentials of Repairing the Body.

International Standard Book Number (ISBN): 978-0-9906029-3-4
Printed in the United States of America

Contents

Appendices

Indices

Translator's Introduction to *Zhèng Tǐ Lèi Yào* (Categorized Essentials of Repairing the Body)

Zhèng Tǐ Lèi Yào (Categorized Essentials of Repairing the Body) was written by Xuē Jǐ during the *Míng* dynasty (薛己《正體類要》明). A summary of information regarding Xuē Jǐ and this book is given in the table below.

Xuē Jǐ 薛己, the Author	
family name	Xuē 薛
míng-name*	Jǐ 己
zì-name	Xīnfǔ 新甫
hào-name	Lìzhāi 立齋
dynasty	Míng 明
hometown	Wújùn 吳郡 (Sūzhōu region)
born	1487
died	1559
Xuē Jǐ's age at death	72
Xuē Jǐ's age when this book was published	61
year this book was published	1548

*Chinese males traditionally took a number of names over the course of their lives. To an outsider, this can be very confusing. The *míng*-name (名) is given by parents shortly after the child is born. The *zì*-name (字) is sometimes called a courtesy name. This was used by peers on formal occasions and in writing. A *hào*-name (號) is a self-selected pen name.

Xuē Jǐ's Life, Achievements, and Philosophy

For more details on the author and his impact on medicine, please see the Translator's Introduction to *Outline of Female Medicine*.[1] What follows is a summary.

---

1. *Nǚ Kē Cuò Yào*《女科撮要》by Xuē Jǐ, translated by Lorraine Wilcox and published by The Chinese Medicine Database in 2016.

Xuē Jǐ grew up with a medical lineage in his family and also rose through the ranks of the Imperial Academy of Medicine. He himself treated members of the imperial family including even the Emperor. Eventually, Xuē became the Commissioner of the Nánjīng Imperial Academy of Medicine. He later resigned from office and returned to his hometown to practice medicine and write.

Xuē Jǐ wrote prolifically. He authored or edited and annotated at least sixteen books. Some were officially published in his government capacity while others were published after he retired. Xuē was interested in a broad array of topics, including internal medicine, external medicine, diseases of the mouth and teeth, female disorders, and pediatrics. Xuē Jǐ added an extensive number of his own case studies to the various books he wrote and annotated.

Retrospectively, Xuē Jǐ is said to have been one of the founders of the School of Warm Supplementation.[2] The main theory is that since yáng is life, strengthening the patient with warming herbs is generally necessary. If the body's yáng qì is strong, the patient can recover from most diseases without attacking the disease. Xuē, emphasized both the spleen and kidneys. By analyzing the prescriptions in a number of books, it can be seen that Xuē's most commonly used formulas (including variations) are:

Bǔ Zhōng Yì Qì Tāng 補中益氣湯
Bā Wèi Wán 八味丸
Liù Wèi Dì Huáng Wán 六味地黃丸
Sì Wù Tāng 四物湯
Sì Jūn Zǐ Tāng 四君子湯
Liù Jūn Zǐ Tāng 六君子湯
Bā Zhēn Tāng 八珍湯
Shí Quán Dà Bǔ Tāng 十全大補湯
Guī Pí Tāng 歸脾湯
Xiǎo Chái Hú Tāng 小柴胡湯

These formulas are all still commonly-used today, so reading Xuē's cases can guide us in our modern clinical practice. The cases can expand our understanding of formulas we already use. While some formulas in this book may be inappropriate today due to the inclusion of endangered species or toxic ingredients, much of Xuē's medicine is still appropriate in the modern clinic.

---

2. *Wēn bǔ xué pài* 溫補學派.

Since Xuē Jǐ favored supplementation (especially warm supplementation), he was disinclined to see a condition as excess; if an excess was acknowledged, it was usually viewed as the branch, with deficiency as the root. He therefore rarely used purely draining formulas and never used attacking formulas. Even in conditions that appear to be excess, Xuē preferred to use supplementing formulas, adding draining herbs as needed.

Xuē Jǐ generally favored using mild herbs over a longer period of time. If his cases are truthfully reported, Xuē cured serious injuries without causing side effects. His philosophy was that if the patient's original qì is strong, he or she could recover. Therefore, he avoided any quick fixes that could harm the patient's strength, but his treatment was slower acting.

Xuē Jǐ included many case histories to illustrate his treatments. This book contains 84 of his own cases. Case studies are important because we can see the doctor's clinical thought in action. Essays on a topic often provide insight to a theory, but when case after case is provided, the application of the theory becomes clear.

Later doctors frequently criticize earlier ones. Xuē Jǐ was criticized for not following classical thought, for relying excessively on warm supplementation, and for being a jack of all trades, master of none since he wrote books on many departments of medicine.

External medicine was Xuē Jǐ's specialty, and the topic of this book, the treatment of traumatic injury, is closely related.

About This Book, *Zhèng Tǐ Lèi Yào*

Correcting or repairing the body (*zhèng tǐ* 正體 or *zhěng tǐ* 整體) is a specialty of medicine concerned with correcting or mending broken bones, dislocations, wounds, or other kinds of physical injury. It is equivalent to traumatology (*shāng kē* 傷科). As described in the original preface to the book, this specialty was sometimes looked down upon because it involves hands-on techniques such as bone-setting, physical manipulations, lancing of infected wounds, blood-letting, and so forth. Even though he specialized in external medicine and trauma, Xuē Jǐ, as an imperial medical officer, must have still retained relatively high status. However, it is notable that in this book, there is no mention of the author himself setting a broken bone or reducing a dislocated joint. Patients came to him after seeing a bone-setter (for example, see cases 3-13, 3-16, and 3-26). Xuē did, however, lance and let blood. It is not clear whether he performed any amputations or simply prescribed for them to be done when needed.

Because the author did not set bones or reduce dislocation, there are no directions for these techniques in *Zhèng Tǐ Lèi Yào*. Such descriptions can be found in many other books on traumatology. However, the lack of descriptions for bone-setting techniques here should not be a big loss for the modern reader because:

▶ A manual technique cannot be learned from a text alone. It is essential to have a teacher in clinic to learn such techniques properly.
▶ There are different techniques for manipulations to treat such injuries, and the ones described in ancient books often are not considered the best ones today.
▶ Most of us will be treating patients with traumatic injuries after they have left the emergency department of the hospital. Chinese medicine will usually only be consulted for follow-up care in modern times. In this respect, our role is similar to that of Xuē Jǐ. Like Doctor Xuē, we will not treat patients right after the trauma. Our care will come once their bones have been set or dislocations have been reduced. Our role will be to ensure that long-term healing progresses smoothly so the patient can return to his or her life as it was before the injury.

One of the major concerns in ancient times was that wounds could easily fester (become infected, in modern terms). Today, we tend to think that a course of antibiotics can prevent or cure any serious infections. However, antibiotics have begun to fail us. Many multi-drug resistant bacteria now surround us and iatrogenic infections are a real threat. Recently, scientists in England followed a recipe from a thousand-year-old Anglo Saxon medical book and found that it kills MRSA quite effectively.[3] The abstract reads, in part:

> The remedy repeatedly killed established *S. aureus* biofilms in an *in vitro* model of soft tissue infection and killed methicillin-resistant *S. aureus* (MRSA) in a mouse chronic wound model. While the remedy contained several ingredients that are individually known to have some antibacterial activity, full efficacy required the combined action of several ingredients, highlighting the scholarship of premodern doctors and the potential of ancient texts as a source of new antimicrobial agents.

There is no reason why this type of ability would not also be found in various ancient Chinese remedies. Perhaps some of the formulas for internal or external use in *Zhèng Tǐ Lèi Yào* may also be effective for modern nightmares such as 'flesh-eating bacteria' (necrotizing fasciitis) or MRSA, etc.

Zhèng Tǐ Lèi Yào is organized into five sections. The first goes over general treatment methods for various aspects of injury: from pain, to bleeding, to tetanus and everything in between. The second section describes the treatment of patients after a beating or caning.[4] The third is the treatment of wounds and injuries from falls, injuries from metal (such as knife wounds), and even frostbite. The fourth part is for burns and scalds. The second, third, and fourth parts contain case after case to illustrate the clinical application of the methods described in part one. The final part, all of Volume 2, contains seventy-five formulas or procedures to treat such conditions.

The reader should note that a passage of text may not mention the original injury. It should be assumed that the condition discussed comes from an injury of the type mentioned in the heading or sub-heading for that passage. The first

---

3. A 1,000-Year-Old Antimicrobial Remedy with Antistaphylococcal Activity, mBio. 2015 Jul-Aug; 6(4): e01129-15. http://www.ncbi.nlm.nih.gov/pmc/articles/ PMC4542191/, viewed on 11/26/2015.
4. Caning is a type of corporal punishment that was used by the justice system, employers, and within the family. The cane is made of rattan. It is thinner than the walking stick type of cane, but can cause serious damage and scarring that remains for the rest of the person's life. Caning was common in the past, in the east or west. It is still used today as corporeal punishment in a few countries.

section has sub-headings for rib-side pain, abdominal pain, vomiting, etc. They describe treatment of these conditions when they occur after an injury and do not discuss more generalized conditions of rib-side pain, abdominal pain, vomiting, and so forth. Some of the cases also fail to name the specific injury, but one should assume that trauma that led to the symptoms mentioned. For example, a case may begin with rib-side pain and other symptoms, but if it is within the section for beatings, one must assume that the rib-side pain came from a beating. This is another indication that Xuē was concerned with long-term healing and not simply the emergency care given immediately after the trauma occurred.

The concept of patient confidentiality did not exist during the *Míng* dynasty. It is interesting to note that none of the cases give the patient's name in the second section, which describes injuries from beatings and canings. However, Xuē often identified the patient in the third section, where many of the injuries were from falling off a horse or other types of accidental injury. This is likely due to a class difference between these two types of patients. Scholars and government officials were less likely to be injured in a brawl or receive corporal punishment (or if they did, they would not want to be identified). Falling off a horse was a more respectable way to receive an injury.

Patients died in nine of these 84 cases. In eight of them, it was because the patient took herbal formulas from other doctors. In some cases, this delayed proper treatment from Xuē but in others, the patient did not trust Xuē's abilities, was impatient for faster results, or was afraid of lancing or amputation. Of course, Xuē was able to choose which cases to include, so we do not find any failures that he attributed to himself. In a couple of cases, the patient did not respond to Xuē's initial treatment or even worsened, but the Xuē decided that 'the strength of the medicine had not arrived yet.' His response was to continue with the same treatment, and even to use a higher dose of *fù zǐ*. In these cases, the patient then improved.

Treatment Methods

Besides using internal formulas (pills, powders, and decoctions), Xuē Jĭ gave at least nineteen formulas that could be used externally. These included ointments, plasters, pastes, washes, dry powders to be sprinkled on a moist area, and so forth. He also used external procedures such as ironing (for example, stir-frying scallions until hot and applying them to the affected site), bleeding (for blood stasis), lancing (for pus), and amputation or removal of dead flesh. Sometimes an enema was suggested for constipation that accompanied an injury. If a patient was dazed or unconscious, herbs were poured into his mouth.

In this book, Xuē Jĭ recommends or performs *biān*-lancing a number of times but the details of the method are not described. His directions for lancing are given in *Lì Yáng Jī Yào* 《 癘瘍機要 》 (Key Essentials of Epidemic Sores) and *Wài Kē Shū Yào* 《 外科樞要 》 (Pivotal Essentials for External Medicine). Between these two books, Xuē said *biān*-lancing was indicated for blood stasis, wind toxins,[5] seasonal toxins, cinnabar toxins, or clove sores (*dīng chuāng*); there may be red threads running away from the site. Here are the directions for performing the technique from *Wài Kē Shū Yào*:

用細磁器擊碎，取有鋒芒者一塊，以箸一根，劈開頭尖夾之，用線縛定 。

Smash something made of fine porcelain and select a sharp shard. Split the end of a chopstick open, jam the sharp shard into the opening, and bind it on securely with thread.

兩手指輕撮箸，梢令磁芒正對患處懸寸許；再用箸一根，頻擊箸頭，令毒血遇刺皆出 。毒入腹膨脹者難治 。

With two fingers, gently hold the end of the chopstick so the porcelain shard directly faces the affected site, suspended about a cùn above it. Then

---

5. A common physical manifestation of toxins is pus; the *biān*-lancing removes the pus and hence most of the toxins.

use another chopstick to repeatedly tap the end of the first chopstick, pricking the affected site to make all the toxins and blood come out.

In *Zhèng Tǐ Lèi Yào*, every time Xuē Jǐ wrote to needle (*zhēn* 針) or prick (*cì* 刺) the affected site, his intention was to remove pus or blood stasis. While it is possible that Xuē used some type of metal needle for this as well as a porcelain shard, he never mentioned acupuncture or moxibustion[6] in this book.

The Healing Process

The process of wound healing has a number of steps, which can be summarized as follows[7]:

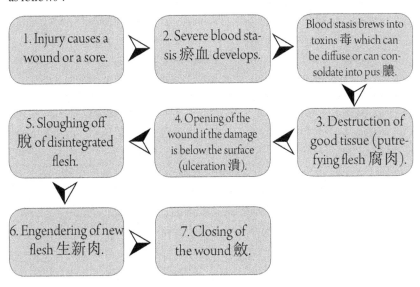

1. Injury causes a wound or a sore.

2. Severe blood stasis 瘀血 develops.

Blood stasis brews into toxins 毒 which can be diffuse or can consolidate into pus 膿.

5. Sloughing off 脫 of disintegrated flesh.

4. Opening of the wound if the damage is below the surface (ulceration 潰).

3. Destruction of good tissue (putrefying flesh 腐肉).

6. Engendering of new flesh 生新肉.

7. Closing of the wound 斂.

If the wound is minor, not all of these steps need occur. However, certain stages of this process may be inevitable in a particular case and problems can occur at any of these steps. Therefore, in different cases, Xuē describes the inability

---

6. In one case (3-37), Xuē ironed a patient in the region of the umbilicus with hot mugwort, but surprisingly, there is no burning of mugwort in this book.
7. Modern texts on traumatology or external medicine may have differences. This outline is based on analysis of Xuē Jǐ's writings. It should be noted that there are different schools of thought on external medicine, and Western biomedicine has also influenced modern texts.

to form pus, or to ulcerate, or to grow new flesh, or for the wound to close up. In most cases, he felt that failure to complete a stage was due to deficiency. If the body is strong, the healing should progress smoothly. Therefore, Xuē most often prescribed supplementing herbs for internal use and herbs or procedures to treat the branch for external use.

What can go wrong in the healing process?

▶ Blood stasis that doesn't disperse or flesh that has been destroyed may fester and develop toxins. In beginning stages, the toxins are diffuse in the flesh but they can consolidate into pus.[8] When diffuse, toxins can spread into good neighboring flesh. When toxins condense into pus, at least they are more localized.

▶ Pus is not necessarily a bad sign. If it is thick (膿稠), it is part of the healing process. Forming thick pus means the toxins have all condensed into one place and can then be let out of the body. If it is clear, thin, and watery (膿水清稀) or foul (膿穢), healing is not progressing properly. Sometimes it is a poor sign when pus does not form at all. All of these conditions are attributed, at least in part, to the patient's deficiency, so the body is unable to respond.

▶ Red lively 紅活 flesh in the affected site is good, showing that qì and blood can flow through the region. Dull 黯 or dark 黑色 color flesh is a bad sign. If qì and blood cannot flow through the region, it cannot heal and festering can expand into healthy adjacent areas.

▶ Flesh that has been badly injured needs to break down and slough off or be removed. If the injury is under intact skin (perhaps after a caning), it needs to open up to the outside or ulcerate 潰. If it ulcerates to the inside instead, the festering spreads within the body and can kill the patient. If the wound opens to the outside, healing can progress. When this kind of damage is under the surface, the treatment is to lance and/or bleed it, and then to remove the pus, blood stasis, and disintegrating flesh.

---

8. Perhaps this is parallel to the difference between yángmíng channel pattern and yángmíng organ pattern. In the channel pattern, heat evils are diffuse throughout the body (similar to diffuse toxins). In the organ pattern, the evils have condensed into stool (similar to toxins consolidating into pus). Obviously, different treatment strategies are necessary during the two stages. When evils are diffuse, one counteracts them. When consolidated, one removes them from the body.

▶ If blood stasis from trauma is inside the abdomen, it might be let out by descending (promoting a bowel movement) in a strong patient, but this method is too draining for a deficient patient. Xuē Jǐ occasionally descended such cases, but often thought the patient was too weak. Unlike many other doctors, Xuē preferred to transform the stasis internally.

▶ Drawing out the interior (or internal expression 托裏) is the treatment method of pushing toxins (including pus) outward from the inside of the body by supplementing right qì. Xuē used formulas to draw out the interior relatively often.

▶ Once the blood stasis and toxins are removed from the affected site, new flesh needs to form and then the wound needs to close up. If qì or blood is weak, these final stages of healing may not occur. Just as qì holds the lower orifices and the so-called pores shut, and also holds blood in the vessels, qì also promotes the closing of a wound. If the patient is deficient, closing cannot occur.

One should also note that other factors may affect the healing process. For example, a number of cases involve liver fire due to anger. The anger heats up the liver; since the liver stores blood, the blood becomes hot. This causes an increase in bleeding or deficiency of liver blood. Diet, alcohol use, bedroom activities, taxation (working too much), or worry can also affect the healing process by causing deficiency or the build-up of heat.

For the Reader

The formulas are indexed as follows:

Examples	Letter	Formula Number	Meaning
F-4	F = Formula	4	The fourth recipe given (F-4 *Bā Zhēn Tāng*).
UF-5	UF = Unlisted Formula that the author used but did not give the recipe,	5	The fifth recipe given in the translator's appendix of unlisted formulas at the end of the book (UF-5 *Tiáo Zhōng Yì Qì Tāng*).

UFx-2	UFx = Unlisted Formula that the author did not use (taken by the patient without being prescribed by the author)	2	The second recipe given in the translator's appendix of unlisted and unused formulas at the end of the book (UFx-2 *Tòu Gǔ Dān*).

Note that the indications listed for formulas are usually focused on the topic of the book – treatment of traumatic injuries. A formula often has many more indications than are listed here, but Xuē usually limited his description of usage to the ones that were relevant.

A Few Terms

I will not make an extensive glossary here, but a few terms warrant discussion. Some years ago I stuck closely to the terminology developed by Nigel Wiseman. As my understanding grows, I now sometimes deviate from it. One reason is that terms have been used differently in different time periods and by different authors. The terms below do not have good English equivalents or Xuē Jǐ used them in his own way.

Ulcerate (*kuì* 潰): to ulcerate, fester, open, or rupture. The original meaning was a river overflowing its banks or the bursting of a dike or dam. In disease and wound healing, this is when damaged flesh with blood stasis or pus opens to the outside of the body. However, internal ulceration (the festering area opening to the interior) is a very bad turn of events as the toxins and decay can then spread to the internal organs. When a wound or sore ulcerates to the outside, the toxins and decay can leave the body and recovery can progress, so ulceration is not a bad sign. However, if ulceration becomes chronic and does not heal, recovery is delayed.

As a treatment method, *ulcerate* can mean to expel pus (*pái nóng* 排膿). A variety of methods are used to make sores ulcerate and expel pus, including internal prescriptions, external application, and lancing.

Descending (*xià* 下): This word is used in many ways in general speech and in medical contexts. Its meanings include down, below, under, lower, to descend, to move downward, to swallow, to come out from below, the lower body, and so forth. In this text it is translated differently according to the context. The problem comes when discussing the treatment principle of *xià* 下. This is often translated as *purge* (which means to cleanse, not to descend). Wiseman uses *precipitate* (precipitation descends from above, but English speakers have difficulty seeing the connection). Bensky discusses *downward-draining* herbs (probably the best rendering but cumbersome). There is no perfect translation.

While the treatment principle of descending (*xià*) tends to result in a bowel movement, the emphasis is on descending something substantial that is unwanted and letting it out through the lower orifices. Besides stool, the term is also used for blood stasis in the uterus, inducing labor, retention of placenta, and so forth.

Channel (*jīng* 經): The author often attributed a symptom to a problem in a channel, even though it seems organ-related to the modern practitioner. He used this term in the same way as *entering channels* for herbs. An herb that enters the spleen channel may actually treat the spleen organ. A symptom attributed to the liver channel, for example, may actually be related to the internal part of the channel that goes to the liver itself.

Original qì (*yuán qì* 元氣): While pronounced the same, do not confuse it with source qì (*yuán qì* 原氣). Original qì is used more or less as a synonym for right qì (*zhèng qì* 正氣), the sum of everything that promotes health in the body. Xuē Jǐ valued supporting original qì far more than dispersing evils.

Finally

One more item to discuss is that in this book, qì or blood deficiency can result in fevers or heat conditions. In modern times we tend to think of qì and blood deficiency as contributing to cold conditions, or at least not making heat. To understand Xuē Jǐ's theories please refer to the writings of Lǐ Dōngyuán 李東垣 and Zhū Dānxī 朱丹溪, much of which have been translated into English.

Warning: Please note that some of the formulas in this book are not appropriate for use today. They may contain herbs that are now considered toxic or unclean. They may contain herbs from endangered species. In the sections that give the recipes for the formulas, the translator has tried to footnote all instances of herbs that can no longer be used. However, it is possible that some herbs to be avoided have been missed. While most of the formulas in this book are still clinically relevant, it is the practitioner's responsibility to determine whether they are appropriate for use in a specific case, or if they are appropriate for use at all in the modern world.

This book describes serious injuries and their aftermath from the point of view of a sixteenth century doctor. Today, there are different standards of care that must be followed. Much of the information is still very useful clinically but other parts are only of historical interest. The reader must decide what is appropriate and not go beyond what is reasonable, safe, or legal. The reader should be able to assess the degree of injury and make proper referrals when necessary. In many cases, Western medicine should be used for initial care or when various warning signs are present. Infections, shock, blood loss, broken bones, and so forth should be taken seriously. If you are not up to the task, refer appropriately and quickly.

Weights and Measures

During the *Míng* dynasty, when this was written, the following were the standard:

one liǎng	一兩	37.30 grams
one qián	一錢	3.73 grams
one fēn	一分	0.37 grams
one gě	一合	59.68 grams
one jīn	一斤	596.8 grams
one shēng	一升	1073.7 ml
one chǐ	一尺	31.10 cm
one cùn	一寸	3.11 cm

Acknowledgments

It takes many people to make a book ready for publication. In recent years, my go-to person for questions has been and still is Yue Lu. She is knowledgeable and patient with me and has devoted a lot of time to making this book understandable. Jerome Jiang is the best when it comes to understanding ancient medical culture and the formal writings of government officials. Micah Arsham read portions of the book and gave useful suggestions. Finally, my publisher and editor is Jonathan Schell. Besides making the book look nice by laying it out and designing the cover, he puts up with my argumentative nature without getting angry at me. This is no small task. My deepest thanks and gratitude go to these people.

序
Preface

世恆言：醫有十三科。科自專門，各守師說，少能相通者，其大較然也。然諸科方論，作者相繼，纂輯不遺，而正體科獨無其書。豈非接復之功，妙在手法；而按揣之勞，率鄙為粗工，而莫之講歟。

For generations, it has commonly been said that there are thirteen departments of medicine.[1] Departments have their own specialties, each following the master's teachings. Few are able to communicate with each other; the majority of them are this way. Although all the various departments have their formulas and discourses compiled by authors one after another to ensure that nothing is lost, only the department of repairing the body does not have its own writings. Isn't the skill of rejoining and restoring [sinews and bones] displayed in the subtlety of manual techniques? But the labor of pressing and probing is often scorned as unskilled work, so no one discusses it.

昔我毅皇帝因馬逸傷，諸尚藥以非世業莫能治，獨吾蘇徐通政鎮侍藥奏效，聖體如初，而徐亦由此遭際，擢官至九列，子孫世以其術仕醫垣。此其所系，豈小小者而可以弗講也！

In the past, none of the imperial doctors were able to treat our Emperor Yì,[2] when he was injured after a horse got loose. This was because they had not learned [the skills of repairing the body] in their hereditary practice. The only one who served him herbs that were effective was our Xú Zhèn from Sūzhōu, from the Office of Transmission; the saintly body [of the Emperor recovered

---

1. During the *Míng* dynasty, one list of the thirteen departments of medicine included treating adults, children, women, skin conditions, acupuncture-moxibustion, eyes, mouth and teeth, throat, bone-setting, cold damage, metal and arrow wounds, *ànmó*-manipulation and massage, and incantations.
2. This is a posthumous name for Emperor Zhèngdé who ruled from 1505-1521.

so that he] was like before. From this encounter, Xú also advanced to the ninth rank of officials and for generations his descendants used his techniques while serving in the imperial medical services. How is this a small thing that is unneccessary to discuss!?

且肢體損於外，則氣血傷於內，榮衛有所不貫，臟腑由之不和，豈可純任手法，而不求之脈理，審其虛實，以施補瀉哉？

Furthermore, when the body is harmed on the outside, qì and blood are injured on the inside, so there are places through which *yíng* and *wèi* cannot pass. The *zàngfǔ*-organs become disharmonious from this. How could one trust manual techniques alone, and not seek out the principles of medicine, examining the patient's deficiency or excess in order to carry out supplementation and draining!?

太史公有言：人之所病，病疾多，醫之所病，病道少。吾以為患在不能貫而通之耳。秦越人過琅琊即為帶下醫，過洛陽即為耳目痹醫，入咸陽即為小兒醫。此雖隨俗為變，豈非其道固無所不貫哉！

In the words of the Grand Historian[3]: People have many types of diseases, but doctors have few methods of treatment. I take this to refer to the suffering that exists from the inability to practice and then master medicine. Qín Yuèrén[4] went to Lángyá and became a women's doctor; he went to Luòyáng and was an ear, eye, and *bì*-obstruction specialist; he entered Xiányáng and became a pediatrician. He followed the local customs and changed this way. How could there be anything in his *dào*-path that he could not practice!

---

3. Sīmǎ Qiān who wrote *Shǐ Jì* 司馬遷《史記》. This quote is found in Volume 105, in the biography of Biǎn Què 扁鵲.

4. Qín Yuèrén 秦越人 is another name for Biǎn Què 扁鵲. This sentence is also paraphrased from Volume 105 of *Shǐ Jì*.

立齋薛先生，以癰疽承家，而諸科無所不治。嘗病正體家言
獨有未備，間取諸身所治驗，捻而集之，為《正體類要》若
干卷，極變析微，可謂詳且盡矣。而處方立論，決生定死，
固不出諸科之外也。然則學者，又豈病道之少乎？

Doctor Xuē Lìzhāi has taken abscesses as his specialty, but there is nothing he
does not treat in any of the departments of medicine. He was concerned that
the words of specialists in repairing the body alone have not been comprehen-
sively explained. In the interval, he has chosen cases from his own treatment
experience and collected them to become the volumes of *Zhèng Tǐ Lèi Yào*
(Categorized Essentials of Repairing the Body). In this book, he has pro-
foundly analyzed disease changes; one can say that he has exhausted the details
for now. And in setting forth his views on prescriptions or on determining
[the prognosis of] life or death, this certainly does not go beyond the various
departments of medicine. That being so, then how are there 'few methods of
treatment'[5] for people who are learning!?

先生嘗著《外科樞要》，余既為之序以刻矣。將復刻是書，
備一家言，余仰其用心之勤，乃復為綴數語卷首，使後世知
先生之術，固無所不通，而未嘗不出於一也，學人其勿以專
門自誘哉。

Doctor Xuē wrote *Wài Kē Shū Yào* (Pivotal Essentials for External Medicine);
I wrote a preface for it when it was printed. I shall again print this book, which
contains the comprehensive words of one specialist. I admire his diligent hard
work, so I again composed several sentences for the beginning of the volume
to let later generations know of the doctor's skill. Certainly, there is nothing
he fails to understand and it never comes from anywhere other than the one
source. People who are learning should not focus on only one specialty.

---

5. This refers back to the statement in the previous paragraph that "people have many
types of diseases, but doctors have few methods of treatment."

先生名己，字新甫，官位出處，詳《外科樞要序》中，茲不
更列。

The doctor's *míng*-name is Jǐ and his *zì*-name is Xīnfǔ. The details of his official position and background are in the Preface to *Wài Kē Shū Yào*, so I'll not list them again here.[6]

前進士禮部主事陸師道著
Written by former Metropolitan Graduate (*jìn shì*) and
Secretary at the Ministry of Rites, Lù Shīdào

---

6. This paragraph should give details of Xuē Jǐ's names and positions, but is very terse. See the trasnslator's introduction for more information.

Volume 1

《正體類要·上卷·正體主治大法》
1. Fundamental Methods Governing Treatment when Repairing the Body

一、脅肋脹痛：若大便通和，喘咳吐痰者，肝火侮肺也，用小柴胡湯加青皮、山梔清之。若胸腹脹痛，大便不通，喘咳吐血者，瘀血停滯也，用當歸導滯散通之。

▶ **Rib-side distention and pain[7]:**

◊ If defecation is harmonious but there is panting, cough, and spitting phlegm, it is liver fire insulting the lungs; clear it using F-2 *Xiǎo Chái Hú Tāng*[8] adding *qīng pí* and *zhī zǐ*.[9]

◊ If there is chest and abdominal distention and pain and defecation is obstructed, with panting, cough, and spitting blood, it is blood stasis that collects and stagnates; free it using F-44 *Dāng Guī Dǎo Zhì Sǎn*.

---

7. In this and the sections below, the assumption is that the original condition was due to traumatic injury, not pathology of the internal organs. However, problems in healing occur when the organs are unable to perform their appropriate functions. So in this section, the rib-side distention and pain may have appeared after a beating or falling off a horse.

8. The formulas are described in Volume 2. 'F' indicates that this is a formula and '2' means that it is the second formula given in Volume 2. The rest of the formulas are numbered using the same method.

9. The author used the name *shān zhī* 山梔, but most English readers are more familiar with *zhī zǐ* 梔子. Both refer to the same herb. I have used more familiar terms in the English text for a number of herbs. For example, the author wrote *dān pí* 丹皮 but I changed the English to *mǔ dān pí* 牡丹皮. No changes have been made in the Chinese characters.

28

《內經》云：肝藏血，脾統血。蓋肝屬木，生火侮土，肝火既燬，肝血必傷，脾氣必虛。宜先清肝養血，則瘀血不致凝滯，肌肉不致遍潰；次壯脾健胃，則瘀血易潰，新肉易生。若行克伐，則虛者益虛，滯者益滯，禍不旋踵矣。

Nèi Jīng says: The liver stores blood; the spleen controls blood.[10] The liver belongs to wood so it engenders fire and insults earth. When liver fire has been blazing, liver blood will be injured and spleen qì will become deficient. One should first clear the liver and nourish blood; then it will not result in blood stasis with congealing stagnation and it will not result in ulcerations developing throughout the muscles and flesh. Next, invigorate the spleen and fortify the stomach; then blood stasis easily ulcerates and new flesh easily grows.[11] If one acts to subdue and cut down [by using attacking herbs], this will increase the deficiency in a deficient person and increase the stagnation in a stagnant person. Disaster is not far behind.

一、肚腹作痛：或大便不通，按之痛甚，瘀血在內也，用加味承氣湯下之。既下而痛不止，按之仍痛，瘀血未盡也，用加味四物湯補而行之。若腹痛按之不痛，血氣傷也，用四物湯加參、耆、白朮，補而和之。若下而胸脅反痛，肝血傷也，用四君、芎、歸補之。既下而發熱，陰血傷也，用四物、參、朮補之。既下而惡寒，陽氣傷也，用十全大補湯補之。既下而惡寒發熱，氣血俱傷也，用八珍湯補之。既下而欲嘔，胃氣傷也，用六君、當歸補之。既下而泄瀉，脾腎傷也，用六君、肉果、破故紙補之。若下後，手足俱冷，昏憒出汗，陽氣虛寒也，急用參附湯。吐瀉手足俱冷，指甲青者，脾腎虛寒之甚也，急用大劑參附湯。口噤手撒，遺尿痰盛，唇青體冷者，虛極之壞症也，急投大劑參附湯，多有得生者。

---

10. "The spleen controls blood" does not occur in *Sù Wèn* or *Líng Shū* although the concept may be stated using other words. "The liver stores blood" is found in *Sù Wèn*, Chapter 62 and *Líng Shū*, Chapter 8.
11. In healthy healing, wounds with significant blood stasis need to open up (ulcerate) to let the stasis or toxins out; only then can new flesh grow. If healing is delayed, the wound may not ulcerate, or it may ulcerate without growing new flesh.

► **Bellyache:**

◊ If defecation is obstructed and pain is severe when pressed, blood stasis is present internally; descend it [promote a bowel movement] using F-10 *Jiā Wèi Chéng Qì Tāng*.

◊ If the pain does not stop after being descended [a bowel movement has occurred] and there is still pain when pressed, the blood stasis is not completely removed; supplement and move it using F-8a *Jiā Wèi Sì Wù Tāng*.

◊ If abdominal pain stops hurting when pressed, blood and qì are injured; supplement and harmonize them using F-8 *Sì Wù Tāng* adding *rén shēn*, *huáng qí*, and *bái zhú*.

◊ If, contrary to expectations, the chest and rib-sides become painful after being descended, liver blood is injured; return and supplement it using F-1 *Sì Jūn Zǐ Tāng* with *chuān xiōng*.

◊ If fever develops after being descended, yīn and blood are injured; supplement them using F-8 *Sì Wù Tāng* with *rén shēn* and *bái zhú*.

◊ If there is aversion to cold after being descended, yáng qì is injured; supplement it using F-16 *Shí Quán Dà Bǔ Tāng*.

◊ If there is aversion to cold and fever after being descended, qì and blood are both injured; supplement them using F-4 *Bā Zhēn Tāng*.

◊ If there is a desire to vomit after being descended, stomach qì is injured; supplement it using F-34 *Liù Jūn Zǐ Tāng* with *dāng guī*.

◊ If there is diarrhea after being descended, the spleen and kidneys are injured; supplement them using F-34 *Liù Jūn Zǐ Tāng* with *ròu guǒ* (nutmeg) and *pò gù zhǐ*.

◊ If the hands and feet are all cold and the patient is dazed and sweats after being descended, yáng qì is deficient and cold; quickly use F-17 *Shēn Fù Tāng*.

◊ When there is vomiting and diarrhea with cold hands and feet and *qīng*-green fingernails, the spleen and kidneys are extremely deficient and cold; quickly use a large dose of F-17 *Shēn Fù Tāng*.

◊ If there are clenched jaws, limp hands, incontinence of urine, abundant phlegm, *qīng*-green lips, and coldness of the body, it is a disintegrating condition of extreme deficiency; many will be able to live if they are quickly given a large dose of F-17 *Shēn Fù Tāng*.

一、肌肉間作痛：營衛之氣滯也，用復元通氣散。筋骨作
痛，肝腎之氣傷也，用六味地黃丸。內傷下血作痛，脾胃之
氣虛也，用補中益氣湯。外傷出血作痛，脾肺之氣虛也，用
八珍湯。大凡下血不止，脾胃之氣脫也，吐瀉不食，脾胃之
氣敗也，苟預為調補脾胃，則無此患矣。

► **Pain within the muscles and flesh:**

◊ For stagnation of *yíng* and *wèi* qì, use F-37 *Fù Yuán Tōng Qì Sǎn.*

◊ Pain of the sinews and bones means injury to the liver and kidneys; use F-29 *Liù Wèi Dì Huáng Wán.*

◊ Internal injury with bleeding from below and pain means spleen and stomach qì deficiency; use F-23 *Bǔ Zhōng Yì Qì Tāng.*

◊ External injury with bleeding and pain means spleen and lung qì deficiency; use F-4 *Bā Zhēn Tāng.*

◊ Generally speaking, incessant bleeding from below means spleen and stomach qì desertion; vomiting and diarrhea with no intake of food means conquered spleen and stomach qì; if the patient has attuned and supplemented the spleen and stomach beforehand,[12] he will not suffer this.

一、作痛：若痛至四五日不減，或至一二日方痛，欲作膿
也，用托裏散。若以指按下復起，膿已成也，刺去其膿，痛
自止。若頭痛時作時止，氣血虛也，痛而兼眩屬痰也，當生
肝血補脾氣。

► **Pain:**

◊ If pain does not decrease within four or five days, or if it is one or two days before pain occurs, pus is about to develop; use F-42 *Tuō Lǐ Sǎn.*

◊ If the affected site is pressed down with a finger and it rises up again, it has already developed pus; prick it to remove the pus and the pain will stop.

◊ If there is headache off and on, qì and blood are deficient. Simultaneous pain and dizziness belongs to phlegm; one should engender liver blood and supplement spleen qì.

---

12. *Supplementing beforehand* means doing it at the time of the initial injury so that these problems are not encountered later in the healing process.

一、青腫不潰：用補中益氣湯以補氣。腫黯不消，用加味逍
遙散以散血。若焮腫脹痛，瘀血作膿也，以八珍加白芷托
之。若膿潰而反痛，氣血虛也，以十全大補湯補之。若骨骱
接而復脫，肝腎虛也，用地黃丸。腫不消，青不退，氣血虛
也，內用八珍湯，外用蔥熨法，則瘀血自散，腫痛自消。若
行血破血，則脾胃愈虛，運氣愈滯。若敷貼涼藥，則瘀血益
凝，內腐益深，致難收拾。

▶ *Qīng*-green swellings [contusions] that do not ulcerate:

◊ Supplement qì using F-23 *Bǔ Zhōng Yì Qì Tāng*.

◊ When the swelling is dull-colored and does not disperse, dissipate blood using UF-1 *Jiā Wèi Xiāo Yáo Sǎn*.[13]

◊ If there is scorching swelling and distenting pain, blood stasis is developing into pus; draw it out using F-4 *Bā Zhēn Tāng* adding *bái zhǐ*.

◊ If pus is discharged, but contrary to expectations, it is painful, qì and blood are deficient; supplement them using F-16 *Shí Quán Dà Bǔ Tāng*.

◊ If the bones and sockets have been rejoined but repeatedly dislocate, the liver and kidneys are deficient; use F-29 *Dì Huáng Wán*.

◊ When swelling does not disperse and the *qīng*-green color does not recede, qì and blood are deficient; internally use F-4 *Bā Zhēn Tāng* and externally use F-3 Scallion Ironing Method. Then the blood stasis will dissipate and the swelling and pain will disperse without any further intervention.

▪ If you move blood or break blood, the spleen and stomach will become more deficient and the transportation of qì more stagnant.

▪ If you apply cooling herbs externally, blood stasis will congeal even more and internal putrefaction will move deeper; the result will be a condition that is difficult to repair.

一、發熱：若出血過多，或膿潰之後脈洪大而虛，重按全
無，此陰虛發熱也，用當歸補血湯。脈沉微，按之軟弱，此
陰盛發躁也，用四君、薑、附。若發熱煩躁，肉瞤筋惕，亡

---

13. Formulas that have UF as a preface were mentioned in the text but the recipe was not given in Volume 2. The recipes for these formulas may be found in the appendices. Formulas with UF were prescribed by the author. Formulas with UFx were mentioned but not prescribed by the author; they were often said to be used mistakenly.

血也，用聖愈湯。如汗不止，血脫也，用獨參湯。其血脫脈
實，汗後脈躁者難治，細小者易治。《外臺秘要》云：陰盛
發躁，欲坐井中，用附子四逆湯加蔥白。王太仆先生云：凡
熱來復去，晝見夜伏，夜見晝伏，不時而動者，名曰無火，
此無根之虛火也。

▶ **Fever:**

◊ If a patient who has bled excessively or after discharge of pus has a pulse
that is surging and large but deficient and nothing is felt when it is strongly
pressed, the fever is due to yīn deficiency; use F-14 *Dāng Guī Bǔ Xuè Tāng*.

◊ If the pulse is sunken and faint, and it is soft and weak when pressed, it is
yīn exuberance with agitation; use F-1 *Sì Jūn Zǐ Tāng* with ginger and *fù zǐ*.

◊ If there is fever with vexation, agitation, twitching flesh, and jerking
sinews, it is collapse of blood; use F-15 *Shèng Yù Tāng*.

◊ If sweating does not stop and blood is deserting, use F-11 *Dú Shēn Tāng*.

◊ Someone is difficult to treat if blood has deserted but the pulse is excessive or if the pulse is agitated after sweating; if the pulse is fine or small, the
patient is easy to treat.

◊ *Wài Tái Mì Yào* states: For someone with yīn exuberance, agitation, and
a desire to sit in a well, use UF-2 *Fù Zǐ Sì Nì Tāng* adding *cōng bái*.

◊ Doctor Wáng Tàipū[14] wrote: Whenever heat comes and goes again,
appearing in the day but subsiding at night, or coming out at night but
subsiding in the day, stirring at irregular times, this is called *lacking fire*, this
is unrooted deficiency fire.

一、作嘔：若因痛甚，或因克伐而傷胃者，用四君、當歸、
半夏、生薑。或因忿怒而肝傷者，用小柴胡湯加山梔、茯
苓。若因痰火盛，用二陳、薑炒黃連、山梔。若因胃氣虛，
用補中益氣湯、生薑、半夏。若出血過多，或因潰後，用六
君子湯加當歸。

---

14. This is another name for Wáng Bīng 王冰. He wrote this in his commentary on *Sù
Wèn*, Chapter 74 although it is paraphrased here.

▸ **Nausea and Vomiting:**

◊ If it is due to severe pain or injury to the stomach due the use of herbs that subdue and cut down, use F-1 *Sì Jūn Zǐ Tāng* with *dāng guī*, *bàn xià*, and *shēng jiāng*.

◊ Or if it is due to anger and rage injuring the liver, use F-2 *Xiǎo Chái Hú Tāng* adding *zhī zǐ* and *fú líng*.

◊ If due to abundance of phlegm-fire, use UF-3 *Èr Chén Tāng* plus *huáng lián* stir-fried with ginger and *zhī zǐ*.

◊ If due to stomach qì deficiency, use F-23 *Bǔ Zhōng Yì Qì Tāng* with *shēng jiāng* and *bàn xià*.

◊ If bleeding excessively or after ulceration [of a sore or wound], use F-34 *Liù Jūn Zǐ Tāng* adding *dāng guī*.

一、喘咳：若出血過多，面黑胸脹；或胸膈痛而發喘者，乃氣虛血乘於肺也，急用二味參蘇飲。若咳血衄血者，乃氣逆血蘊於肺也，急用十味參蘇飲加山梔、芩、連、蘇木。

▸ **Panting and Cough:**

◊ If the patient is bleeding excessively with a dark face and chest distention; or if pain of the chest and diaphragm leads to panting, it is blood taking advantage of qì deficiency in the lungs; quickly use F-7 *Èr Wèi Shēn Sū Yǐn*.

◊ If the patient is coughing blood with spontaneous external bleeding,[15] it is qì counterflow with blood amassing in the lungs; quickly use F-6 *Shí Wèi Shēn Sū Yǐn* adding *zhī zǐ*, *huáng qín*, *huáng lián*, and *sū mù*.

一、作渴：若因出血過多，用四物參朮湯；不應，用人參、黃耆以補氣，當歸、熟地以養血。若因潰後，用八珍湯。若因胃熱傷津液，用竹葉黃耆湯。胃虛津液不足，用補中益氣湯。胃火熾盛，用竹葉石膏湯。若煩熱作渴，小便淋瀝，乃腎經虛熱，非地黃丸不能救。

---

15. This term usually means nosebleeds but can mean other forms of external bleeding.

▶ **Thirst:**

◊ If it is due to excessive bleeding, use F-8 *Sì Wù Shēn Zhú Tāng*.[16]

▪ If he does not respond, supplement qì using *rén shēn* and *huáng qí* and nourish blood with *dāng guī* and *shú dì*.

◊ If thirst occurs after ulceration [of a sore or wound], use F-4 *Bā Zhēn Tāng*.

◊ If due to stomach heat injuring *jīnyè*-fluids, use F-25 *Zhú Yè Huáng Qí Tāng*.

◊ For stomach deficiency with insufficient *jīnyè*-fluids, use F-23 *Bǔ Zhōng Yì Qì Tāng*.

◊ For stomach fire blazing vigorously, use F-26 *Zhú Yè Shí Gāo Tāng*.

◊ If there is vexation, heat, thirst, and rough urination with *lín*-dribbling, it is deficiency heat of the kidney channel; he cannot be rescued without F-29 *Dì Huáng Wán*.

一、出血：若患處或諸竅出者，肝火熾盛，血熱錯經而妄行也，用加味逍遙散，清熱養血。若中氣虛弱，血無所附而妄行，用加味四君子湯，補益中氣。或元氣內脫，不能攝血，用獨參湯加炮薑以回陽；如不應，急加附子。或血蘊於內而嘔血，用四物加柴胡、黃芩。

▶ **Bleeding:**

◊ If the patient is bleeding at the affected site or from the various orifices, liver fire blazes vigorously and causes blood heat to disorder the channels and move recklessly; clear heat and nourish blood using UF-1 *Jiā Wèi Xiāo Yáo Sǎn*.

◊ If central qì is deficient and weak, blood has nothing to enclose it so it moves recklessly; supplement and boost central qì using UF-4 *Jiā Wèi Sì Jūn Zǐ Tāng*.

◊ Or original qì deserts internally with inability to contain the blood; return yáng using F-11 *Dú Shēn Tāng* plus *pào jiāng*.

▪ If he does not respond, quickly add *fù zǐ*.

◊ Or blood amasses internally or and there is vomiting of blood; use F-8 *Sì Wù Tāng* adding *chái hú* and *huáng qín*.

---

16. *Sì Wù Shēn Zhú Tāng* is F-8 *Sì Wù Tāng* plus *rén shēn* and *bái zhú*.

凡傷損勞碌怒氣，肚腹脹悶，誤服大黃等藥傷經絡，則為吐
血、衄血、便血、尿血；傷陰絡，則為血積、血塊、肌肉青
黯。此臟腑虧損，經隧失職，急補脾肺，亦有生者。但患者
不司此理，不用此法，惜哉！

Whenever injured by taxation or anger, the belly becomes distended with a
feeling of oppression. When herbs such as *dà huáng* are mistakenly taken, it
injures the channels and *luò*-networks and becomes conditions such as spitting
blood, nosebleeds, bloody stool, or bloody urine; when there is injury to the
yīn *luò*-networks, it becomes blood *jī*-accumulations, blood *kuài*-lumps, and
dull *qīng*-green muscles and flesh. This indicates enfeebled *zàngfǔ*-organs while
the channel-tunnels neglect their duties. If one quickly supplements the spleen
and lungs, the patient might still live. But if the patient does not attend to this
theory and does not use this method, it is a pity!

一、手足損傷：若元氣虛弱，或不戒房勞，或妄行攻伐，致
死肉上延；或腐而不痛，黑而不脫者，當大補元氣，庶可保
生。若手足節骱斷去者，無妨。骨斷筋連，不急剪去。若侵
及好肉則不治。若預為調補脾氣，則無此患。大凡膿瘀肉燃
者，即針之而投托裏散。或口噤遺尿而似破傷風者，急用十
全大補湯加附子，多有生者。

▶ **Injury to the hands and feet:**

◊ If original qì is deficient and weak; or one does not guard against
bedroom taxation;[17] or recklessly enacts treatment to attack and cut down,
it results in dead flesh extending upward or putrefaction without pain but
with blackening [of flesh] that is not sloughed off; one should strongly
supplement original qì. You can ensure life in many patients.

◊ If the joint sockets of the hands and feet are broken, there is no hin-
drance to healing. If the bone is broken but the sinews still connect it, do
not be quick to amputate.

◊ If [dead flesh or putrefaction] invades into good flesh, it cannot be
treated.

---

17. Bedroom taxation (*fáng láo* 房勞) is exhaustion due to excessive sexual activity
with loss of *jīng*-essence.

- If one attunes and supplements spleen qì beforehand,[18] the patient will not suffer this.

◊ Generally speaking, in someone with pus, stasis, and scorching flesh, needle it and give F-42 *Tuō Lǐ Sǎn*.[19]

◊ Or for clenched jaw with incontinence of urine when this appears to be tetanus (*pò shāng fēng*), quickly use F-16 *Shí Quán Dà Bǔ Tāng* adding *fù zǐ*; many will live.

一、腐肉不潰：或惡寒而不潰，用補中益氣湯。發熱而不潰，用八珍湯。若因克伐而不潰者，用六君子湯加當歸。其外皮堅硬不潰者，內火蒸炙也，內服八珍湯，外塗當歸膏。其死肉不能潰，或新肉不能生而致死者，皆失於不預補脾胃也。

▶ **Putrefying flesh that does not ulcerate:**

◊ Perhaps there is aversion to cold and no ulceration; use F-23 *Bǔ Zhōng Yì Qì Tāng*.

◊ For fever without ulceration, use F-4 *Bā Zhēn Tāng*.

◊ If it does not ulcerate due to the [mistaken] use of herbs that subdue and cut down, use F-34 *Liù Jūn Zǐ Tāng* adding *dāng guī*.

◊ If the skin is hard with no external ulceration, and fire is steaming and roasting on the inside, internally take F-4 *Bā Zhēn Tāng* and externally smear on F-41 *Dāng Guī Gāo*.

◊ All cases of death as a result of dead flesh that is unable to ulcerate or new flesh that is unable to grow are lost due to the mistake of failing to supplement the spleen and stomach in advance.

一、新肉不生：若患處夭白，脾氣虛也，用六君、芎、歸。患處緋紅，陰血虛也，用四物、參、朮。若惡寒發熱，氣血虛也，用十全大補湯。膿稀白而不生者，脾肺氣虛也，用補

---

18. One should supplement at the time of the initial injury to prevent necrosis, according to the author.

19. Here *scorching flesh* means a burning sensation in the flesh, inflammation due to infection in modern terms. *Needling* refers to letting blood for stasis or lancing an area that has pus.

中益氣湯。膿稀赤而不生者，心脾血虛也，用東垣聖愈湯。
寒熱而不生者，肝火動也，用加味逍遙散。晡熱而不生，肝
血虛也，用八珍、牡丹皮。食少體倦而不生，脾胃氣虛也，
用六君子湯。膿穢而不生者，元氣內傷也，用補中益氣湯。
如夏月，用調中益氣湯。作瀉用清暑益氣湯。秋令作瀉，用
清燥湯。

► **New flesh does not grow:**

◊ If the affected site is deathly white, spleen qì is deficient; use F-34 *Liù Jūn Zǐ Tāng* with *chuān xiōng* and *dāng guī*.

◊ If the affected site is crimson, yīn and blood are deficient; use F-8 *Sì Wù Tāng* with *rén shēn* and *bái zhú*.

◊ If there is aversion to cold and fever, qì and blood are deficient; use F-16 *Shí Quán Dà Bǔ Tāng*.

◊ If there is thin white pus and flesh does not grow, spleen and lung qì are deficient; use F-23 *Bǔ Zhōng Yì Qì Tāng*.

◊ If there is thin red pus and flesh does not grow, heart and spleen blood are deficient; use Lǐ Dōngyuán's F-15 *Shèng Yù Tāng*.[20]

◊ If there are [sensations of] cold and heat and flesh does not grow, liver fire is stirring; use UF-1 *Jiā Wèi Xiāo Yáo Sǎn*.

◊ If there is late afternoon fever and flesh does not grow, liver blood is deficient; use F-4 *Bā Zhēn Tāng* with *mǔ dān pí*.

◊ If there is decreased food intake, the body is weary, and flesh does not grow, spleen and stomach qì are deficient; use F-34 *Liù Jūn Zǐ Tāng*.

◊ If there is foul pus and flesh does not grow, original qì is injured internally; use F-23 *Bǔ Zhōng Yì Qì Tāng*.

◊ If it is during the summer, use UF-5 *Tiáo Zhōng Yì Qì Tāng*.

■ If there is diarrhea, use UF-6 *Qīng Shǔ Yì Qì Tāng*.

◊ If there is diarrhea during the autumn, use F-19 *Qīng Zào Tāng*.

一、重傷昏憒者：急灌以獨參湯。雖內瘀血切不可下，急用
花蕊石散，內化之，恐因瀉而亡陰也。若元氣虛甚者，尤

---

20. Lǐ Dōngyuán 李東垣 (1180-1251) was one of the Four Great Masters of the *Jīn-Yuán* dynasties and the author of *Pí Wèi Lùn* 《脾胃論》 (Discussion of the Spleen and Stomach). Xuē Jǐ tended to favor his formulas and theories of treatment.

不可下，亦用以前散化之。凡瘀血在內，大小便不通，用大
黃、朴硝。血凝而不下者，急用木香、肉桂末二三錢，以熟
酒調灌服，血下乃生。如怯弱之人，用硝、黃，須加肉桂、
木香同煎，假其熱，以行其寒也。

► **Dazed after a serious injury:**

◊ Quickly pour in F-11 *Dú Shēn Tāng.*[21]

◊ Even if there is blood stasis inside, be sure not to descend [promote a bowel movement] the patient;[22] quickly use F-45 *Huā Ruǐ Shí Sǎn* to transform the stasis internally. Descending risks causing diarrhea and collapse of yīn.

■ If original qì is extremely deficient, you especially cannot descend the patient; still use the above powder (F-45 *Huā Ruǐ Shí Sǎn*) to transform the stasis.

◊ Whenever blood stasis is present inside and urination and defecation are obstructed, use *dà huáng* and *pò xiāo*. If congealed blood does not descend, quickly use two or three *qián* (7.46 - 11.19 grams) of *mù xiāng* and *ròu guì* powder. Mix it with aged liquor and pour it in. The blood will descend and he will live. If the person is physically weak, you must add *ròu guì* and *mù xiāng* when using *pò xiāo* and *dà huáng*. Boil them together, borrowing their heat[23] to move and activate the coldness [of *pò xiāo* and *dà huáng*].

一、大便秘結：若大腸血虛火熾者，用四物湯送潤腸丸，或
以豬膽汁導之。若腎虛火燥者，用六味地黃丸。腸胃氣虛，
用補中益氣湯。

► **Constipation:**

◊ If large intestine blood is deficient with fire blazing, swallow F-13 *Rùn Cháng Wán* using F-8 *Sì Wù Tāng*, or use pig bile[24] as an enema.

---

21. Pouring in (*guàn* 灌) is used for an unconscious patient. The herbal powder or decoction is poured into the person's mouth or maybe into his nose.
22. Descending herbs have been commonly used for blood stasis inside the abdomen.
23. This means the hot nature of *mù xiāng* and *ròu guì*, not the temperature of the liquid.
24. Pig bile clears heat, moistens dryness, and is used to treat constipation as well as

◊ If the kidneys are deficient with fire and dryness, use F-29 *Liù Wèi Dì Huáng Wán.*

◊ If the intestines and stomach are qì deficient, use F-23 *Bǔ Zhōng Yì Qì Tāng.*

一、傷損症用黑羊皮者，蓋羊性熱，能補氣也。若杖瘡傷甚，內肉已壞，欲其潰者貼之，成膿固速。苟內非補劑壯其根本，毒氣不無內侵。外非砭刺，泄其瘀穢，良肉不無傷壞者。受刑輕，外皮破傷者，但宜當歸膏敷貼，更服四物、芩、連、柴胡、山梔、白朮、茯苓。又丁痂不結，傷肉不潰，死血自散，腫痛自消。若概行罨貼，則醞釀瘀毒矣。

► **The use of black goat skin for injuries:**

◊ The nature of goat is hot and it supplements qì.

◊ If wounds from a caning are severe and the flesh inside has already disintegrated, stick it on when the wounds are about to ulcerate; they are sure to develop pus quickly.[25]

▪ If supplementing prescriptions are not used internally to invigorate the root, toxic qì will not fail to invade internally.

▪ If it is not pricked with a *biān*-lance externally to drain stasis and foulness, good flesh will not fail to be injured and disintegrate.

◊ If the physical punishment received was light and the skin was broken and injured externally, it is appropriate to stick on F-41 *Dāng Guī Gāo* [instead of black goat skin]; further take F-8 *Sì Wù Tāng* with *huáng qín, huáng lián, chái hú, zhī zǐ, bái zhú,* and *fú líng.* Then scabs will not form, injured flesh will not ulcerate, dead blood will automatically scatter, and swelling and pain will automatically disperse. If you stick black goat skin on indiscriminately [in light cases like this], it will brew stasis and toxins.

---

internal heat diseases, jaundice, cough, red eyes, and so forth. Pig bile may be taken internally in decoctions, pills, or with powders. Externally, it can be spread on a site, used in eye drops, or as an enema. Xuē tended to use it for constipation, often as an enema, although there are recipes for decocting pig bile with honey and taking it internally for bound up dry stool. Xuē mentioned using it to make F-13 *Rùn Cháng Wán,* below.

25. Developing pus is a healthy response at certain stages of wound healing. It means that the body is strong enough to respond to the injury and toxins are being pushed out of the body. See the translator's introduction.

一、跳躍捶胸閃挫，舉重勞役恚怒，而胸腹痛悶，喜手摸者，肝火傷脾也，用四君、柴胡、山梔。畏手摸者，肝經血滯也，用四物、柴胡、山梔、桃仁、紅花。若胸脅作痛，飲食少思，肝脾氣傷也，用四君、芎、歸。若胸腹不利，食少無寐，脾氣鬱結也，用加味歸脾湯。若痰氣不利，脾肺氣滯也，用二陳、白朮、芎、歸、梔子、青皮。若咬牙發搐，肝旺脾虛也，用小柴胡湯、川芎、山梔、天麻、鉤藤鉤。或用風藥，則肝血益傷，肝火愈熾。若用大黃等藥，內傷陰絡，反致下血。少壯者必為痼疾，老弱者多致不起。以上若胸脅作痛，發熱晡熱，肝經血傷也，用加味逍遙散。

▶ **Pain and oppression of the chest and abdomen from leaping, beating one's chest, sprains, lifting weights, forced labor, or becoming enraged:**

◊ If he likes it to be touched, liver fire is injuring the spleen; use F-1 *Sì Jūn Zǐ Tāng* with *chái hú* and *zhī zǐ*.

◊ If he fears being touched, it is blood stagnation of the liver channel; use F-8 *Sì Wù Tāng* with *chái hú, zhī zǐ, táo rén,* and *hóng huā*.

◊ If the chest and rib-sides are painful with little thought of food and drink, liver and spleen qì are injured; use F-1 *Sì Jūn Zǐ Tāng* with *chuān xiōng* and *dāng guī*.

◊ If the chest and abdomen are inhibited with decreased food intake and insomnia, it is binding constraint of spleen qì; use F-12a *Jiā Wèi Guī Pí Tāng*.

◊ If phlegm and qì inhibit the chest and abdomen, spleen and lung qì are stagnant; use UF-3 *Èr Chén Tāng* with *bái zhú, chuān xiōng, dāng guī, zhī zǐ,* and *qīng pí*.

◊ If the patient clenches his teeth and twitches, the liver is at peak strength but the spleen is deficient; use F-2 *Xiǎo Chái Hú Tāng* with *chuān xiōng, zhī zǐ, tiān má,* and *gōu téng gōu*.

◊ Perhaps the use of herbs to treat wind has increased the injury to liver blood, so liver fire blazes hotter. If *dà huáng* and similar herbs are used, it injures the yīn *luò*-networks internally, so contrary to expectations, there will be bloody stool. The young and vigorous will develop obstinate disease; it will result in death for many old and weak people.

◊ In the above, if there is chest and rib-side pain, fever, and late afternoon fever, it is injury to the blood of the liver channel; use UF-1 *Jiā Wèi Xiāo Yáo Sǎn*.

一、破傷風：河間云：風症善行數變，入臟甚速，死生在反掌之間，宜急分表裏虛實而治之。

► **Tetanus**[26]:

Liú Héjiān said: Wind conditions tend to move and mutate frequently; they enter the *zàng*-organs very rapidly. Life and death occurs within the space of turning over the hand [very easily and rapidly]. It is appropriate to quickly determine whether it is exterior or interior, deficiency or excess, and then treat it.

邪在表者，則筋脈拘急，時或寒熱，筋惕搐搦，脈浮弦，用羌活防風湯散之。在半表半裏者，則頭微汗，身無汗，用羌活湯和之。傳入裏者，舌強口噤，項背反張，筋惕搐搦，痰涎壅盛，胸腹滿悶，便溺閉赤，時或汗出，脈洪數而弦，以大芎黃湯導之。既下而汗仍出，表虛也，以白朮防風湯補之，不時灌以粥飲為善。前云乃氣虛未損之法也。若膿血太泄，陽隨陰散，氣血俱虛，而類前症者，悉宜大補脾胃，切忌祛風之藥。

◊ When these evils are in the exterior, the sinews and vessels have hypertonicity, now and then there are [sensations of] cold and heat, the sinews jerk and convulse, and the pulse is floating and bowstring; dissipate it using F-60 *Qiāng Huó Fáng Fēng Tāng*.

◊ When it is half exterior and half interior, the head sweats a little but the body does not sweat; harmonize it using F-63 *Qiāng Huó Tāng*.

◊ If it is transmitted into the interior, the tongue is stiff, the jaw is clenched, the nape and back arch backwards, and the sinews jerk and convulse. This

---

26. *Pò shāng fēng* 破傷風 (tetanus) is also called *lockjaw*. It occurs when wind evils enter a wound or sore. It follows a specific course and has a number of symptoms, including tetany (see the next heading).

is abundance of phlegm-drool congesting with fullness and oppression of the chest and abdomen, constipation, red urine, sweating now and then, and the pulse is surging, rapid, and bowstring; lead it out using F-65 *Dà Xiōng Huáng Tāng*.

◊ If the patient was descended[27] but is still sweating, this means it is exterior deficiency; supplement him using F-66 *Bái Zhú Fáng Fēng Tāng*. It is good to frequently pour in rice porridge drink (*zhōu yǐn*). The previous item discusses the method for a patient whose qì has not been harmed.

◊ If pus and blood drain excessively, yáng follows them and yīn scatters; there is deficiency of both qì and blood and it resembles the previous condition. It is completely appropriate to strongly supplement the spleen and stomach; by all means avoid herbs to dispel wind.

一、發痙：仲景云：諸痙項強，皆屬於溫。又云：太陽病，發汗太多，致痙風病。下之則痙復發，汗則拘急。瘡家發汗則痙，是汗下重亡津液所致。

► **Tetany[28]:**

Zhāng Zhòngjǐng said: All tetany with rigid nape corresponds to warmth. He also said: In tàiyáng disease, excessive sweating causes tetany wind disease. If you descend it [promote a bowel movement], tetany relapses; if you promote sweating, hypertonicity occurs. When people who suffer sores or wounds are made to sweat, there is tetany; the reason is that sweating and descending doubly cause collapse of *jīnyè*-fluids.

有汗而不惡寒曰柔痙，以風能散氣也，宜白朮湯加桂心、黃耆。無汗而惡寒曰剛痙，以寒能澀血也，宜葛根湯。皆氣血內傷，筋無所營，而變非風也。杖瘡及勞傷氣血而變者，當補氣血；未應，用獨參湯；手足冷加桂、附，緩則不救。

---

27. Descending is the treatment method that is most often carried out by inducing a bowel movement. Here the author is referring to the previous item - F-65 *Dà Xiōng Huáng Tāng* descends.

28. *Jìng* 痙 (tetany) signifies severe spasms including neck rigidity, arched-back rigidity, clenched jaws, and convulsions. Tetany is seen in different diseases, incuding tetanus. In children, it is called *fright wind*.

◊ If there is sweating and no aversion to cold, it is called *soft tetany*; it uses the ability of wind to scatter qì. It is appropriate to use F-67 *Bái Zhú Tāng* adding *guì xīn* and *huáng qí*.

◊ If there is no sweating and there is aversion to cold, it is called *hard tetany* because cold roughens the flow of blood. It is appropriate to use UF-7 *Gé Gēn Tāng*.

◊ If qì and blood are both injured on the interior, the sinews have nothing to nourish them, so it mutates into wind stroke.

◊ When wounds from caning and taxation injure qì and blood and then mutuate into tetany, you should supplement qì and blood.

- If the patient doesn't respond, use F-11 *Dú Shēn Tāng.*
- For cold hands and feet, add cinnamon and *fù zǐ.*
- When you are late, the patient cannot be rescued.

《正體類要 · 上卷 · 撲傷之症治驗》
2. Treatment Experience Regarding Symptoms of Injury from a Beating

血脫煩躁
Blood Desertion with Vexation and Agitation

2-1 有一患者，兩脅脹悶，欲咳不咳，口覺血腥，遍身臀腿
脹痛，倦怠不食，煩渴脈大。此血脫煩躁也，與童便酒及砭
患處，出死血糜肉甚多。忽發熱煩躁汗出，投以獨參湯三劑
少止，又用補氣血、清肝火之藥數劑，飲食稍進。後用獨參
湯間服，諸症悉退，飲食頓加，但不能多寐，以歸脾湯加山
梔、竹茹，四劑而熟睡。因勞心遂煩渴自汗，脈大無力，以
當歸補血湯二劑而安；又以十全大補去川芎加麥門、五味、
牡丹、地骨、麻黃根、炒浮麥，數劑而汗止，死肉且潰；又
二十餘劑而新肉生。

Both rib-sides of a patient were distended with a feeling of oppression.[29] He had an urge to cough but there was no cough. He perceived that his mouth reeked of blood. His entire body, including his buttocks and legs, were distended and painful. He was fatigued and did not eat. He suffering vexation, thirst, and had a large pulse. This was blood desertion with vexation and agitation. I gave him child's urine[30] and liquor, and then *biān*-lanced the affected site; quite a lot of

---

29. All the cases take place after an injury of the type in the section heading. In this section, the reader should assume that the symptoms of these cases developed after a beating, even if the beating is not mentioned.

30. *Tóng biàn* 童便 (child's urine): This is the urine of a boy who is ten years old or younger. It is salty and cold in nature. Child's urine nourishes yīn, descends fire, cools blood, and scatters stasis. In the past it was used to treat cough, vomiting blood, nosebleeds, postpartum dizziness, and so forth. The best quality is the first urine of the day taken on the morning of the day before the full moon.

dead blood and spoiled flesh came out. He suddenly became feverish with vexation, agitation, and sweating. I gave him three doses of F-11 *Dú Shēn Tāng* and it decreased. I next used several doses of herbs to supplement qì and blood and clear liver fire; he then ate and drank a little. Afterwards I had him take F-11 *Dú Shēn Tāng* at intervals and all the symptoms receded. His eating and drinking immediately increased, but he was unable to sleep much. I used four doses of F-12 *Guī Pí Tāng* adding *zhī zǐ* and *zhú rú* and he slept soundly. Due to taxation of the heart-mind [or worry], he then suffered vexation, thirst, and spontaneous sweating. His pulse was large but forceless. I used two doses of F-14 *Dāng Guī Bǔ Xuè Tāng* and he was peaceful; I then used several doses of F-16 *Shí Quán Dà Bǔ Tāng* removing *chuān xiōng* and adding *mài mén dōng, wǔ wèi zǐ, mǔ dān pí, dì gǔ pí, má huáng gēn,* and stir-fried *fú mài.* The sweating stopped and the dead flesh further ulcerated. After more than twenty additional doses, new flesh grew.

血虛發躁
Blood Deficiency with Agitation

2-2 有一患者，煩躁面赤，口乾作渴，脈洪大，按之如無 。
余曰：此血虛發躁也 。遂以當歸補血湯二劑即止 。後日晡發
熱，更以四物加柴胡 、牡丹 、地骨 、黃柏 、知母治之，熱退
而瘡斂 。

There was a patient with vexation, agitation, red face, dry mouth, and thirst. His pulse was surging and large but it felt like nothing was present when pressed. I said: This is blood deficiency with agitation. I then used two doses of F-14 *Dāng Guī Bǔ Xuè Tāng* and it stopped. Later, he had fevers at sunset, so I further treated him using F-8 *Sì Wù Tāng* adding *chái hú, mǔ dān pí, dì gǔ pí, huáng bǎi,* and *zhī mǔ.* The fevers receded and the wound closed.

東垣云：發熱惡寒，大渴不止，其脈大而無力者，非白虎湯
症，此血虛發躁也，宜用當歸補血湯治之 。裴先生云：肌熱
躁熱，目赤面紅，其脈洪大而虛，此血虛也，若誤用白虎
湯，輕則危，重則斃 。

Lǐ Dōngyuán said that fever with aversion to cold, strong unremitting thirst, and a large but forceless pulse is not a UFx-4 *Bái Hǔ Tāng* condition; it is blood deficiency with agitation. It is appropriate to use F-14 *Dāng Guī Bǔ Xuè Tāng* to treat it. Doctor Péi[31] said: Hot muscles with agitation, fever, red eyes and face, and surging large but deficient pulse is due to blood deficiency; mistakenly using UFx-4 *Bái Hǔ Tāng* is dangerous in mild cases but is an execution in serious cases.

氣虛血熱
Qì Deficiency with Blood Heat

2-3 有一患者，頭額出汗，熱渴氣短，煩躁骨痛，瘀肉不潰，遂割去之，出鮮血，服芩、連之藥益甚，其脈洪大而微。此氣血俱虛，邪火熾盛所致，以四物加參、耆、朮、炙草，少用柴胡、炒芩，二劑頭汗頓止；又加麥門、五味、肉桂，二劑諸症悉退。後用參、耆、歸、朮、炒芍、熟地、麥門、五味，十餘劑瘀血潰而膿水稠矣。但新肉不生，以前藥倍用白朮而斂。

The forehead of a patient was sweating; he was hot and thirsty, suffering shortness of breath, vexation, agitation, and bone pain. The flesh with stasis did not ulcerate, so it was cut out until he bled fresh blood.[32] He took herbs like *huáng qín* and *huáng lián* but the symptoms increased a lot.[33] His pulse was surging and large but faint. The reason was that this was deficiency of both qì and blood with evil fire blazing vigorously. I used two doses of F-8 *Sì Wù Tāng* adding *rén shēn, huáng qí, bái zhú*, and *zhì gān cǎo* plus a little *chái hú* and stir-fried *huáng qín*; the sweating on his head immediately stopped. I then gave him two more

---

31. The identity of this person is currently unknown.
32. After the beating or caning, the blood stasis in this patient's flesh was so severe from the physical trauma that it was incapable of recovery. It was not breaking down and going through the normal healing process Therefore, the dead flesh was removed. From the timeline of the story, it is apparent that another doctor did the surgery.
33. In many cases, the patient has seen another doctor or taken medication on his own before he consulted with Xuē Jǐ. When this is mentioned, Xuē Jǐ rarely, if ever, approved of what was done before.

doses adding *mài mén dōng, wǔ wèi zǐ*, and *ròu guì*, and all the symptoms receded. Afterwards, I used more than ten doses of *rén shēn, huáng qí, dāng guī, bái zhú*, stir-fried *sháo yào, shú dì huáng, mài mén dōng*, and *wǔ wèi zǐ*. The blood stasis ulcerated while the pus-water thickened.[34] However, new flesh did not grow. I used the previous herbs, doubling the dose of *bái zhú*, and the wound subsequently closed up.

瘀血泛注
Flooding and Streaming of Blood Stasis

2-4 有一患者，瘀血流注，腰臀兩足俱黑 。隨飲童便酒，砭出瘀血糜肉，投以小柴胡湯，去半夏加山栀 、芩 、連 、骨碎補，以清肝火；用八珍 、茯苓，以壯脾胃，死肉潰而新肉生 。後瘡復潰，得靜調治，年餘而痊 。

There was a patient with static blood streaming sores.[35] The paravertebral sinews of his lower back and both legs were all black. I let him drink child's urine with liquor and *biān*-lanced the site to remove the blood stasis and spoiled flesh. I gave him F-2 *Xiǎo Chái Hú Tāng* removing *bàn xià* and adding *zhī zǐ, huáng qín, huáng lián*, and *gǔ suì bǔ* to clear liver fire; I used F-4 *Bā Zhēn Tāng* with *fú líng* to invigorate the spleen and stomach. The dead flesh ulcerated and new flesh grew. Afterward, the wound ulcerated again. He obtained calm by attuning and governing himself, and recovered after more than a year.

---

34. Now, because the patient was stronger, the blood stasis in the flesh broke down as it should. Thin pus indicates a weakened body so a thickening of watery pus was a good sign that his body was responding.

35. Streaming sores are sores in deep layers of the body that make toxins which seem to flow through the flesh. *Yū xuè liú zhù* 瘀血流注 (static blood streaming sores) are streaming sores that develop after traumatic injury. They start with hard painful swellings that are red or *qīng*-green in color. The sores eventually become red and scorching hot. As they spread into the adjacent flesh, systemic symptoms develop, such as fever and aversion to to cold. If they heal properly on their own, they develop pus and then ulcerate.

2-5 有一患者，瘀血攻注，陰囊潰而成漏，膿水清稀。所服皆寒涼之劑。診其肝脈短澀，餘脈浮而無力。此肝木受肺金克制，又元氣虛，不能收斂，遂用壯脾胃生氣血之方，元氣少復。後終殁於金旺之日。

There was a patient with static blood attacking and streaming; his yīn sack [scrotum] ulcerated and developed a fistula that exuded clear thin pus-water. The prescriptions he took were all cold and cool. Upon examination, the liver pulse was short and rough; the rest of the pulses were floating and forceless. This was liver wood receiving control and restraint from lung metal; original qì was also deficient and unable to promote contraction of the wound. I then used a formula to invigorate the spleen and stomach and engender qì and blood. Original qì slightly returned. Later, he died on a day when metal was at peak strength.[36]

瘀血作痛
Pain caused by Blood Stasis

2-6 有一患者，腫痛發熱，作渴汗出。余曰：此陰血受傷也。先砭去惡穢，以通壅塞。後用四物、柴胡、黃芩、山梔、丹皮、骨碎補，以清肝火而愈。

There was a patient with swelling, pain, fever, thirst, and sweating. I said: Yīn and blood have received injury. First, I biān-lanced the site, removing the malign foulness in order to free it from congestion. Afterwards, I used F-8 Sì Wù Tāng with chái hú, huáng qín, zhī zǐ, mǔ dān pí, and gǔ suì bǔ to clear liver fire and he then recovered.

---

36. In the Chinese calendar, days are associated with elements according to the ten heavenly stems and the twelve earthly branches. Perhaps both the stem and branch of the day when this patient died belonged to metal, which further pressed on his liver wood.

2-7 有一患者，傷處揉散，惟腫痛不消。余曰：此瘀血在內，
宜急砭之。不從。余以蘿卜自然汁調山梔末敷之，破處以當
歸膏貼之，更服活血之劑而瘥。數年之後，但遇天陰，仍作
癢痛，始知不砭之失。

There was a patient who rubbed his wounded site to dissipate the swelling and
pain but it did not disperse. I said: This is blood stasis on the inside [with no
way out]; it is appropriate to quickly *biān*-lance it. He did not consent. I mixed
the natural juice of *luó bo* (Chinese radish) with *zhī zǐ* powder and applied it. I
stuck F-41 *Dāng Guī Gāo* on the damaged site. He further took a prescription
to enliven blood and recuperated. However, several years later, whenever he
encountered overcast days, he still had itching and pain; only then did he know
the mistake of not *biān*-lancing it.

2-8 有一患者，臀腿黑腫，而反不破，但脹痛重墜，皆以為
內無瘀血，惟敷涼藥，可以止痛。余診其尺脈澀而結。此因
體肥肉濃，瘀血蓄深，刺去即愈，否則內潰，有爛筋傷骨之
患。余入針四寸，漂黑血數升，腫痛遂止。是日發熱惡寒，
煩渴頭痛，此氣血俱虛而然也，以十全大補之劑遂瘥。

There was a patient whose buttocks and legs were black and swollen, but contrary to expectations, the affected sites did not break open; however, they were
distended, painful, swollen, and heavy. He took all this to mean there was no
blood stasis inside. He only applied cooling herbs and was able to stop the pain.
I felt his pulse and the *chǐ* was rough and bound. This was because his fat and
flesh were dense, causing the blood stasis to amass deeply. If pricked to remove
it, he would recover; otherwise it would ulcerate internally and he would suffer
putrefaction of the sinews and injury to the bones.[37] I inserted a needle four
cùn deep and let out several *shēng*[38] of black blood. The swelling and pain then
stopped. That day he had fever, aversion to cold, vexation, thirst, and headache.
It was this way due to deficiency of both qì and blood. I used some doses of
F-16 *Shí Quán Dà Bǔ Tāng* and he then recuperated.

---

37. If the stasis were to ulcerate to the outside of the body, it could heal. If it festered
internally with no way out, it would keep spreading.
38. One *shēng* equaled 1073.7 ml. at the time.

肝火作痛
Pain caused by Liver Fire

2-9 有一患者，瘀血內脹，焮痛發熱，口乾作渴，飲食不甘，四肢倦怠。余曰：此肝火熾盛，脾土受制，故患前症。喜其稟實年壯，第用降火清肝活血之劑而愈。

There was a patient with blood stasis, internal distention, scorching pain, fever, dry mouth, and thirst. Food and drink did not taste sweet and he had fatigued limbs. I said: This is liver fire vigorously blazing while spleen earth is being restrained so you suffer the above symptoms. I was pleased that his endowment [constitution] was full and he was in the prime of life. I only used prescriptions to descend fire, clear the liver, and enliven blood; he then recovered.

肝火忿怒
Liver Fire with Raging Anger

2-10 有一患者，患處脹痛，悲哀忿怒。此厥陰之火，為七情激之而然耳。遂砭去瘀血，以小柴胡湯加山梔、黃連、桔梗而安。後用生肝血、養脾氣之藥，瘡潰而斂。

There was a patient with distention and pain of the affected site, as well as grief and sorrow, indignation and anger. This was fire of juéyīn; the symptoms were this way because the seven emotions aroused the condition. I then *biān*-lanced the affected site to remove the blood stasis and used F-2 *Xiǎo Chái Hú Tāng* adding *zhī zǐ*, *huáng lián*, and *jié gěng*. He was then peaceful. I later used herbs to engender liver blood and nourish spleen qì. The wound ulcerated and then closed up.

肝火脅脹
Liver Fire with Rib-Side Distention

2-11 有一患者，患處脹痛，發熱欲嘔，兩脅熱脹，肝脈洪大。余曰：肝火之症也。但令飲童便，並小柴胡湯加黃連、山梔、歸梢、紅花，諸症果退。

The affected site of a patient was distended and painful. He had fever, desire to vomit, and heat and distention of both rib-sides. His liver pulse was surging and large. I said: This is a condition of liver fire. I made him drink child's urine and at the same time, F-2 *Xiǎo Chái Hú Tāng* adding *huáng lián, zhī zǐ, dāng guī shāo,* and *hóng huā.* As a result, all symptoms receded.

此症若左關脈浮而無力，以手按其腹，反不脹者，此血虛而肝脹也，當以四物、參、苓、青皮、甘草之類治之。若左關脈洪而有力，胸脅脹痛者，按之亦痛，此怒氣傷肝之症也，以小柴胡、芎、歸、青皮、芍藥、桔梗、枳殼主之。

▶ In this condition, if the left *guān* pulse is floating and forceless, and contrary to expectations, the abdomen is not distended when pressed with the hand, this is blood deficiency leading to liver distention;[39] one should treat it using herbs in the category of F-8 *Sì Wù Tāng* with *rén shēn, fú líng, qīng pí,* and *gān cǎo.*

▶ If the left *guān* pulse is surging and forceful with chest and rib-side distention and pain that is still painful when pressed, this is a condition of anger injuring the liver; treatment is governed by the use of F-2 *Xiǎo Chái Hú Tāng* with *chuān xiōng, dāng guī, qīng pí, sháo yào, jié gěng,* and *zhǐ qiào.*

---

39. The translator found this a little hard to follow, so let me rephrase it for the reader. The patient has liver fire and rib-side distention after a beating. One would expect this to be an excess condition, but the pulse shows deficiency. One would also think that the abdomen would be distended and painful at the same time. However, when pressed, there is no distention or pressing makes the abdominal distention better, so this must be deficiency. The author's explanation is that liver blood deficiency has led to the liver fire and rib-side distention.

蓋此症不必論其受責之輕重，問其患處去血之曾否。但被人
扭按甚重，努力恚怒，以傷其氣血，瘀血歸肝，多致前症。
甚則胸脅脹滿，氣逆不通，或血溢口鼻，卒至不救。

Now, in this condition, one need not bother discussing the heaviness of his
punishment; instead ask whether or not blood [stasis] has been removed from
the affected site. However, when a person is violently seized and restrained by
someone and fights hard while enraged, it injures his qì and blood; the result-
ing blood stasis returns to the liver and he often arrives at the above condition.
When serious, there is distention and fullness of the chest and rib-sides, counterflow qì with obstruction, and perhaps blood spills out from the mouth and
nose; it may suddenly reach the point where he cannot be rescued.

肝膽虛症
A Liver-Gallbladder Deficiency Condition

2-12 有一患者，愈後口苦，腰脅脹痛。服補腎行氣等藥不
愈。余按其肝脈浮而無力。此屬肝膽氣血虛而然耳。用參、
耆、歸身、地黃、白朮、麥門、五味，治之而愈。

After recovery, a patient had a bitter mouth with distention and pain of his
lower back and rib-sides. He took herbs to supplement the kidneys, move qì,
and so forth but did not recover. I pressed his liver pulse and found it floating and forceless. This belonged to deficiency of qì and blood in the liver and
gallbladder, so it was this way. I treated him with *rén shēn, huáng qí, dāng guī shēn,
dì huáng, bái zhú, mài mén dōng,* and *wǔ wèi zǐ;* he recovered.

血虛腹痛
Blood Deficiency with Abdominal Pain

2-13 有一患者，杖後服四物、紅花、桃仁、大黃等劑，以逐
瘀血，腹反痛，更服一劑痛益甚，按其腹不痛。余曰：此血

虛也，故喜按而不痛，宜溫補之劑。遂以歸身、白朮、參、
耆、炙草二劑，痛即止。

After being caned, a patient took a dose of F-8 *Sì Wù Tāng* with *hóng huā, táo rén,
dà huáng* and so forth in order to expel blood stasis. Contrary to expectations,
his abdomen became painful. He took another dose and the pain increased
a lot, but when pressed, his abdomen was not painful. I said: This is blood
deficiency so he likes pressing and it is not painful. It is appropriate to use warm
supplementing prescriptions. I then used two doses of *dāng guī shēn, bái zhú, rén
shēn, huáng qí,* and *zhì gān cǎo.* The pain stopped.

氣虛不潰
Qì Deficiency with Inability to Ulcerate

2-14 有一患者，瘀血已去，飲食少思，死肉不潰，用托裏之
藥，膿稍潰而清。此血氣虛也，非大補不可。彼不從。余強
用大補之劑，飲食進而死肉潰，但少寐，以歸脾湯加山梔二
劑而寐。因勞心煩躁作渴，脈浮洪大，以當歸補血湯二劑而
安。

A patient's blood stasis had already been removed [by lancing], but he had little
thought of food and drink and the dead flesh did not ulcerate. He used herbs
for drawing out the interior;[40] clear pus ulcerated [discharged] a little. This was
blood and qì deficiency; without strong supplementation, he could not recover.
He did not agree. I steadfastly used prescriptions for strong supplementation;
he began eating again and the dead flesh ulcerated. However, he slept little so I
used two doses of F-12 *Guī Pí Tāng* adding *zhī zǐ* and he was able to sleep. Due
to taxation of the heart [worry], he had vexation, agitation, and thirst. His pulse
was floating,[41] surging, and large, so I used two doses of F-14 *Dāng Guī Bǔ Xuè
Tāng* and he became peaceful.

---

40. *Tuō lǐ* 托裏 (drawing out the interior): Also translated as *internal expression*. This
is the treatment method of pushing toxins (including their manifestation as pus) outward from the inside of the body by supplementing right qì.
41. Some editions do not have the word *floating.*

寒凝不潰
Congealing Cold with Inability to Ulcerate

2-15 有一患者，受刑太重，外皮傷破，瘀血如注，內肉糜爛
黯腫，上胤胸背，下至足指，昏憒不食。隨以黑羊皮熱貼患
處，灌以童便酒薄粥，更以清肝活血、調氣健脾之劑。神思
稍蘇，始言遍身強痛。又用大劑養血補氣之藥，腫消食進。
時仲冬瘀血凝結，不能潰膿，又用大補之劑，壯其陽氣，其
膿方熟，遂砭去，洞見其骨，塗以當歸膏，及服前藥百餘
劑，肌肉漸生。

There was a patient who had received excessively heavy physical punishment.
Externally, his skin was broken open with blood stasis that seemed to be pouring out, while his flesh inside was reduced to a pulp and was dull and swollen.
The wounds were continuous from his chest and upper back down to his toes.
He was in a daze and did not eat. I then heated black goat skin to stick onto
the affected sites and poured in child's urine, liquor, and thin *zhōu*-porridge.
I further used prescriptions to clear the liver, enliven blood, regulate qì, and
fortify the spleen. His mental state revived a little and he began to speak, saying
his entire body was stiff and painful. I then used a large dose of herbs to nourish
blood and supplement qì. The swelling dispersed and he began to eat. It was
the second month of winter, so the blood stasis congealed and was unable to
ulcerate pus [due to the cold weather]. I then used a prescription to strongly
supplement. It invigorated his yáng qì and the pus ripened. I then *biān*-lanced
the sites to remove the pus. The bone was visible through the cavity. I smeared
on F-41 *Dāng Guī Gāo* and he took more than a hundred doses of the prevous
herbs. The muscles and flesh gradually grew back.

脾虛不斂
Spleen Deficiency with Inability to Close [a Wound]

2-16 有一患者，潰而不斂，以內有熱毒，欲用寒涼之藥。余曰：此血氣俱虛，而不能斂耳，非歸、茯、參、耆之類，培養脾土，則肌肉何由而生？豈可復用寒涼克伐之藥，重損氣血哉！遂用前藥治之而愈。

There was a patient whose wound had ulcerated but did not close up. He took this as internal heat toxins and wanted to use cold and cool herbs. I said: This is deficiency of both blood and qì leading to inability to close up. If we don't use herbs like *dāng guī*, *fú zǐ*, *rén shēn*, and *huáng qí* to bank up the spleen and nourish earth, what can the muscles and flesh use for growth? How can you recover using cold and cool herbs to subdue and cut down, doubling the harm to qì and blood?! I then used the above herbs to treat him and he recovered.

血虛筋攣
Blood Deficiency with Sinew Spasms

2-17 有一患者，腹脹嘔吐眩暈，用柴胡、黃芩、山梔、紫蘇、杏仁、枳殼、桔梗、川芎、當歸、赤芍、紅花、桃仁，四劑而定。後又出血過多，昏憒目黑，用十全大補等藥而蘇。時肌肉潰爛，膿水淋漓，筋攣骨痛。余切其脈浮而澀，沉而弱。此因氣血耗損，不能養筋，筋虛不能束骨，遂用養氣血之藥，治之而愈。

There was a patient with abdominal distension, vomiting, and dizziness. I used four doses of *chái hú*, *huáng qín*, *zhī zǐ*, *zǐ sū yè*, *xìng rén*, *zhǐ qiào*, *jié gěng*, *chuān xiōng*, *dāng guī*, *chì sháo*, *hóng huā*, and *táo rén*; it settled down. Later he bled excessively and was dazed with darkened vision. I used F-16 *Shí Quán Dà Bǔ Tāng* and so forth, and he revived. At the time, his muscles and flesh festered and dripped pus-water; he had hypertonicity of the sinews and bone pain. I felt his pulse and it was floating, rough, sunken, and weak. This was due to consumption of qì and blood with inability to nourish the sinews; the deficient sinews were unable to bind the bones. I then treated him with herbs to nourish qì and blood and he recovered.

腎虛氣逆
Kidney Deficiency with Qì Counterflow

2-18 有一患者，杖瘡愈後，失於調理，頭目不清。服祛風化痰等藥，反眩暈；服牛黃清心丸，又肚腹疼痛，杖痕腫癢，發熱作渴，飲食不思，痰氣上升，以為杖瘡餘毒復作。診左尺脈洪大，按之如無。余曰：此腎經不足，不能攝氣歸源。遂用人參、黃耆、茯苓、陳皮、當歸、川芎、熟地、山藥、山茱萸、五味、麥門、炙草，服之而尋愈。後因勞，熱渴頭痛，倦怠少食，用補中益氣湯加麥門、五味而痊。

After recovering from wounds from a caning, a patient didn't take proper care of himself. His head and eyes were not clear. He took herbs to dispel wind and transform phlegm and so forth, but contrary to expectations, he became dizzy. He took UFx-1 *Niú Huáng Qīng Xīn Wán*; he then got a bellyache and the caning scars swelled and itched. He had fever, thirst, no thought of food and drink, and phlegm and qì moved upward. I took this as a relapse caused by toxins remaining in the wounds from the caning. I felt his pulse; the left *chǐ* was surging and large, but it felt like nothing was present when pressed. I said: This is insufficiency of the kidney channel with inability to absorb qì and return it to the source. I then used *rén shēn, huáng qí, fú líng, chén pí, dāng guī, chuān xiōng, shú dì, shān yào, shān zhū yú, wǔ wèi zǐ, mài mén dōng,* and *zhì gān cǎo.* He took it and moved toward recovery. Later, due to taxation, he had fever, thirst, headache, fatigue, and reduced food intake. I used F-23 *Bǔ Zhōng Yì Qì Tāng* adding *mài mén dōng* and *wǔ wèi zǐ* and he recuperated.

濕熱乘肝
Damp-heat Taking Advantage of the Liver

2-19 有一患者，愈後腿作痛。余意膿血過多，瘡雖愈，肝經血氣尚未充實，而濕熱乘虛也。遂以八珍加牛膝、木瓜、蒼朮、黃柏、防己、炙草以祛濕熱，養陰血，痛漸止。乃去防己、黃柏，服之遂瘳。

After recovery, a patient had leg pain. I thought the discharge of pus and bleed had been excessive. Even though the wounds had recovered, blood and qì of the liver channel had not yet filled in, so damp-heat took advantage of the deficiency. I then used F-4 *Bā Zhēn Tāng* adding *niú xī, mù guā, cāng zhú, huáng bǎi, fáng jǐ,* and *zhì gān cǎo* to dispel damp-heat and nourish yīn and blood. The pain gradually stopped. I then removed *fáng jǐ* and *huáng bǎi*. He took it and was then healed.

肝經鬱火
Constrained Fire of the Liver Channel

2-20 有一患者，瘀血失砭，脹痛煩渴，縱飲涼童便，渴脹頓止；以蘿卜細搗塗之，瘀血漸散。已而患處作癢，仍塗之癢止。後口乾作渴，小腹引陰莖作痛，小便如淋，時出白津。此肝經鬱火也，遂以小柴胡湯加大黃、黃連、山梔飲之，諸症悉退，再用養血等藥而安。夫小腹引陰莖作痛等症，往往誤認為寒症，投以熱劑，則諸竅出血，或二便不通，以及危殆，輕亦損其目矣。

There was a patient who had neglected to *biān*-lance his blood stasis. He had distention, pain, vexation, and thirst. He drank cool child's urine without restraint and the thirst and distention immediately stopped. He smeared finely pounded *luó bo* on the affected site, and the blood stasis gradually dissipated. Shortly after, the affected site began itching; he still smeared it on and the itching stopped. Afterwards, his mouth became dry, he was thirsty, and he had pain radiating from his lower abdomen to his penis. His urination resembled *lín*-dribbling, and sometimes white *jīn*-fluids were discharged. This was constrained fire of the liver channel. I then had him drink F-2 *Xiǎo Chái Hú Tāng* adding *dà huáng, huáng lián,* and *zhī zǐ.* All his symptoms receded. I again used used herbs to nourish blood and so forth, and he was peaceful. Now, pain radiating from the lower abdomen to the penis and similar conditions are often mistakenly seen as cold conditions; when they are given hot prescriptions, the patient bleeds from the various orifices or there is obstruction of urine and stool. This leads to great danger. In mild cases, it still harms the eyes.

痛傷胃嘔
Painful Injury to the Stomach with Vomiting

2-21 有一患者，痛甚發熱，嘔吐少食，胸膈痞滿。用行氣破血之劑益甚，口乾作渴，大便不調，患處色黯。余曰：此痛傷胃氣所致。遂以四君、當歸、炒芩、軟柴、藿香，二劑諸症漸愈；又用大補之劑，潰之而瘳。

There was a patient who had severe pain, fever, vomiting, and reduced food intake as well as *pǐ*-glomus[42] and fullness of the chest and diaphragm. He used prescriptions to move qì and break blood but the symptoms increased a lot, adding dry mouth, thirst, and stool irregulatities. The affected site became dull-colored. I said: This is caused by pain injuring stomach qì. I then used two doses of F-1 *Sì Jūn Zǐ Tāng* with *dāng guī,* stir-fried *huáng qín, ruǎn chái hú,* and *huò xiāng.* All the conditions gradually recovered. I then used prescriptions to strongly supplement. The affected site ulcerated and then healed.

---

42. *Pǐ*-glomus (痞) is a subjective feeling of fullness and obstruction in the abdomen or chest. Nothing is found upon palpation.

藥傷胃嘔
Injury to the Stomach from Medicine with Vomiting

2-22 有一患者，發熱焮痛，服寒涼藥，更加口乾作渴，肚腹亦痛，自以為瘀血，欲下之。余按其肚腹不痛，脈細微而遲，飲食惡寒。此涼藥傷胃而然也，急用六君加芍藥、當歸、炮附子各一錢，服之前症益甚，反加譫語面赤。余意其藥力未至耳。前藥再加附子五分，服之即睡，覺來諸病頓退而安。

There was a patient with fever and scorching pain who took cold and cooling herbs. Even more, he now had dry mouth and thirst, while his belly was also painful. He himself took it to be blood stasis and wanted to descend it [promote a bowel movement]. I pressed his belly and it was not painful. His pulse was fine, faint, and slow. He was averse to cold food and drink. He was this way because cooling herbs had injured his stomach. I quickly used F-34 *Liù Jūn Zǐ Tāng* adding one *qián* (3.73 grams) each of *sháo yào*, *dāng guī*, and blast-fried *fù zǐ*. He took it but the earlier symptoms increased a lot; contrary to expectations, delirious speech and red face were added. I thought that the strength of the medicine had not arrived yet. I used the previous herbs again adding five more *fēn* (1.85 grams) of *fù zǐ*. He took it and then slept; when he woke up, all his diseases immediately receded and he was peaceful.

氣血不損
No Harm to Qì and Blood

2-23 有一患者，瘀血雖去，飲食形氣如故，但熱渴焮痛，膈痞有痰，以小柴胡湯加天花粉、貝母、桔梗、山梔，二劑少愈；又加生地、歸尾、黃芩、柴胡、山梔、花粉而愈。余治百餘人，其杖後血氣不虛者，惟此一人耳，治者審之。

Even though a patient's blood stasis had been removed [by lancing], his eating and drinking, physical body, and qì were unchanged. However, he was hot and thirsty and he had scorching pain and *pǐ*-glomus of the diaphragm with phlegm. I used two doses of F-2 *Xiǎo Chái Hú Tāng* adding *tiān huā fěn, bèi mǔ, jié gěng,* and *zhī zǐ,* and he recovered a little. I then added *shēng dì, dāng guī wěi, huáng qín, chái hú, zhī zǐ,* and *tiān huā fěn* and he recovered. I have treated more than a hundred people after they were caned, but only this one person had no deficiency of blood and qì; those who treat should know about this.

行氣之非
Mistakenly Moving Qì

2-24 有一患者，服行氣之劑，胸痞氣促，食少體倦，色黯膿清。此形氣俱虛之症也。先用六君、桔梗二劑，胸膈氣和；後用補中益氣去升麻，加茯苓、半夏、五味、麥門治之，元氣漸復而愈。若用前劑，戕賊元氣，多致不救。

There was a patient who took a prescription to move qì. He developed chest *pǐ*-glomus, hasty breathing, reduced food intake, weary body, dull color, and clear pus. This was a deficiency condition of both the physical body and qì. First I used two doses of F-34 *Liù Jūn Zǐ Tāng* with *jié gěng,* and the qì of his chest and diaphragm harmonized. Later I treated him using F-23 *Bǔ Zhōng Yì Qì Tāng* removing *shēng má* and adding *fú líng, bàn xià, wǔ wèi zǐ,* and *mài mén dōng.* His original qì gradually returned and he recovered. If the previous prescription [to move qì] is used, it robs original qì, and the result is often that the patient cannot be rescued.

下血之非
Mistakenly Descending Blood

2-25 有一患者，去其患處瘀血，用四物、柴胡、紅花治之，焮痛頓止。但寒熱口乾，飲食少思，用四物、白朮、茯苓、柴胡、黃芩、花粉，四劑寒熱即退。用六君、芎、歸、藿

香，而飲食進。腐肉雖潰，膿水清稀，以前藥倍用參、耆、
歸、朮、茯苓，二十餘劑，腐肉俱潰，膿水漸稠。誤服下藥
一鐘，連瀉四次，患處色黯。喜其脈不洪數，乃以十全大補
倍加肉桂、麥門、五味數劑，肉色紅活，新肉漸生。喜在壯
年，易於調理，又月餘而愈，否則不救。

I removed blood stasis from a patient's affected site and treated him using F-8 *Sì Wù Tāng* with *chái hú* and *hóng huā*. The scorching pain immediately stopped. However, he had [sensations of] cold and heat, dry mouth, and little thought of food and drink. I used four doses of F-8 *Sì Wù Tāng* with *bái zhú, fú líng, chái hú, huáng qín,* and *tiān huā fěn*. The [sensations of] cold and heat receded. I used F-34 *Liù Jūn Zǐ Tāng* with *chuān xiōng, dāng guī,* and *huò xiāng*. He began eating again. Although his putrefying flesh ulcerated, the pus-water was clear and thin. I used more than twenty doses of the previous herbs with double the dose of *rén shēn, huáng qí, dāng guī, bái zhú,* and *fú líng*. The putrefying flesh completely ulcerated and the pus-water gradually thickened. He mistakenly took a cup of descending herbs [to promote a bowel movement]. He then had four continuous incidents of diarrhea and the affected site become dull colored. I was pleased that his pulse was not surging and rapid. I then used several doses of F-16 *Shí Quán Dà Bǔ Tāng* doubling the dose of *ròu guì, mài mén dōng,* and *wǔ wèi zǐ*. His flesh became red and lively-colored and new flesh gradually grew. I was pleased he was in his prime and it was easy for him to take proper care of himself, so he recovered after more than a month. Otherwise [if he were not strong or could not take care of himself] he could not be rescued.

凡杖瘡跌撲之症，患處如有瘀血，止宜砭去，服壯元氣之
劑。蓋其氣已損，切不可再用行氣下血之藥，復損脾胃，則
運氣愈難行達於下，而反為敗症，怯弱者多致夭枉。

Whenever there are wounds from a caning or conditions from tumbles and beatings, if the affected site has blood stasis, the only appropriate thing is to *biān*-lance it to remove the blood stasis and to take prescriptions to invigorate original qì. The qì will have already been harmed, so also be sure to avoid herbs to move qì or descend blood.[43] When you repeatedly harm the spleen and

---

43. *Descend blood* means to make blood stasis in the abdomen leave the body through

stomach, it becomes more difficult for the transporting qì to move freely in the lower body, and contrary to expectations, it becomes a conquering condition. In the physically weak, this often results in premature death.

寒藥之非
Mistaken Use of Cold Medicine

2-26 有一患者腫痛，敷寒涼之藥，欲內消瘀血，反致臀腿俱冷，瘀血，並胸腹痞悶。余急去所敷之藥，以熱童便酒洗患處，服六君、木香、當歸，敷回陽膏，臀腿漸溫；又以前藥去木香，加川芎、藿香、肉桂，四劑瘀血解；乃刺之，更以壯脾胃、養氣血得痊。

A patient with swelling and pain applied cold and cooling herbs [to the affected site]. He wanted to disperse internal blood stasis. Contrary to his expectations, it resulted in coldness of the buttocks and legs, blood stasis, and *pǐ*-glomus and oppression of the chest and abdomen. I quickly removed the herbs he had applied and washed the affected site with hot child's urine and liquor. He took F-34 *Liù Jūn Zǐ Tāng* with *mù xiāng* and *dāng guī* and applied F-35 *Huí Yáng Gāo*. His buttocks and legs gradually warmed up. I then used four doses of the above herbs removing *mù xiāng* and adding *chuān xiōng*, *huò xiāng*, and *ròu guì*; the blood stasis resolved. I then pricked it [to remove the stasis] and further used herbs to invigorate the spleen and stomach and nourish qì and blood. He was able to recuperate.

蓋氣血得溫則行，得寒則凝，寒極生熱，變化為膿。腐潰深大，血氣既敗，肌肉無由而生，欲望其生難矣。

Now, when qì and blood obtain warmth, they move; when they obtain coldness, they congeal. Extreme cold engenders heat and transmutes into pus. The putrid ulceration grows deeper and larger. Blood and qì have been conquered

---

a bowel movement.

so there is nothing from which muscles and flesh can grow, and hope for their growth becomes difficult.

不砭之非
Mistakenly Failing to *Biān*-Lance

2-27 有一患者，發熱煩躁，用四物、黃芩、紅花、軟柴、山梔、花粉，煩熱已清，瘀血深蓄，欲針出之，不從。忽牙關緊急，患處刺痛，始針去膿血即安。用托裏養血，新肉漸長。忽患處瘙癢，此風熱也，用祛風消毒之劑而痊。

There was a patient with fever, vexation, and agitation. I used F-8 *Sì Wù Tāng* with *huáng qín, hóng huā, ruǎn chái hú, zhī zǐ*, and *tiān huā fěn*. The vexation and fever had already cleared but static blood amassed deeply. I wanted to needle [*biān*-lance] to remove it but he did not agree. Suddenly his jaws clenched [tetany] and he had pricking pain at the affected site. I began to needle to remove pus and blood and he grew peaceful. I used herbs to draw out the interior and nourish blood. New flesh gradually grew. Suddenly the affected site began itching; this was wind-heat. I used a prescription to dispel wind and disperse toxins and he recuperated.

不補之非
Mistakenly Failing to Supplement

2-28 有一患者，臀腿脹痛，發熱煩躁，刺去死血，脹痛少寬，熱躁愈甚，此血脫邪火旺而然也。急用獨參湯補之，少愈；又以健脾胃養氣血藥治之，腐肉漸潰遂愈。

There was a patient with distended painful buttocks and legs, fever, vexation, and agitation. Someone pricked it to remove dead blood. The distention and pain was relieved somewhat but the fever and agitation became more severe. It was this way because of blood desertion with evil fire at peak strength. I quickly used F-11 *Dú Shēn Tāng* to supplement him and he recovered a little. I then treated him with herbs to fortify the spleen and stomach and nourish qì and blood. The putrid flesh gradually ulcerated and he then recovered.

大抵此症宜預調補，以顧收斂，切不可伐其氣血，不行補益，以至不能收斂矣。

Generally speaking, for this condition it is appropriate to regulate and supplement in advance,[44] attending to the need to promote contraction. Be sure not to attack the patient's qì and blood; if one doesn't enact supplementing and boosting, the result will be inability of the wound to contract.

破傷風表症
Exterior Pattern of Tetanus

2-29 有一患者，仲夏誤傷手，腰背反張，牙關緊急，脈浮而散，此表症也，遂用羌活防風湯一劑即解。

During the middle month of summer [around June in the Western calendar], a patient accidentally injured his hand. He developed arched-back rigidity and clenched jaws. His pulse was floating and scattered. This was an exterior pattern. I then used one dose of F-60 *Qiāng Huó Fáng Fēng Tāng* and it resolved.

此症若在秋冬腠理致密之時，須用麻黃之類以發汗。此乃暴傷，氣血不損之治法也。

---

44. Xuē Jǐ believed that in serious injury, one should supplement from the beginning of the treatment and not wait for deficiency symptoms to arise. If the body is deficient, the wound cannot heal properly, and Xuē felt that almost without exception, a person would become deficient after a serious injury.

If this pattern occurs in autumn or winter when the *còu lǐ*[45] are closed, herbs like *má huáng* must be used to promote sweating. This is the treatment method for sudden injury when qì and blood are not harmed.

破傷風裏症
Interior Pattern of Tetanus

2-30 有一患者，杖處略破而患此，脈洪大而實，此裏症也。用大芎黃湯一劑，大便微行一次，悉退。若投表藥必死。宜急分表裏虛實而治之，庶無誤矣。

A patient had a slight break [in the skin] on the site where he had been caned and he suffered tetanus. His pulse was surging, large, and excess. This was an interior pattern. I used one dose of F-65 *Dà Xiōng Huáng Tāng*. He had one small bowel movement and the whole condition receded. If he had been given exterior herbs, he would have died. It is appropriate to quickly distinguish exterior and interior, deficiency and excess and then treat it; then there will be no mistakes in numerous cases.

膿內燉類破傷風
Pus Scorching the Interior Category of Tetanus

2-31 有一患者，寒熱口乾，用四物、參、耆、白朮、軟柴、炒芩、麥門、五味，四劑少退，余欲砭去瘀血，不從。後怔忡不寐，飲食少思，牙關牽緊，頭目疼痛，惡寒發熱，此膿內燉也，遂砭去之即安。以八珍、棗仁、麥門、五味，二十劑，前症漸愈。又用前藥及獨參湯，瘀肉漸潰。後因勞又少寐盜汗，以歸脾湯、麥門、五味、遠志而痊。後牙關脹悶，面目燉赤，又似破傷風，仍以為虛，用八珍等藥亦安。

---

45. The term *còu lǐ* 腠理 is often translated as *pores*. Wiseman glosses it as *interstices*.

There was a patient with [sensations of] cold and heat and dry mouth. I used four doses of F-8 *Sì Wù Tāng* with *rén shēn, huáng qí, bái zhú, ruǎn chái hú*, stir-fried *huáng qín, mài mén dōng*, and *wǔ wèi zǐ*; it receded a little. I wanted to *biān*-lance it to remove the blood stasis, but he did not agree. Later, he had fright palpitations, insomnia, little thought of food and drink, clenched jaw, headache, eye pain, aversion to cold, and fever. This was pus scorching the interior. I then *biān*-lanced it to remove the pus and he was peaceful. I used twenty doses of F-4 *Bā Zhēn Tāng* with *suān zǎo rén, mài mén dōng*, and *wǔ wèi zǐ*, and the earlier condition gradually recovered. I then used the above herbs along with F-11 *Dú Shēn Tāng*. The flesh with stasis gradually ulcerated. Later, due to taxation, he was sleeping less and had night sweats. I used F-12 *Guī Pí Tāng* with *mài mén dōng, wǔ wèi zǐ*, and *yuǎn zhì* and he recuperated. Later he had distention and oppression of the jaw and scorching red face and eyes. This again seemed like tetanus. I still took it as deficiency and used herbs like F-4 *Bā Zhēn Tāng* and he again recovered.

膿潰類破傷風
Suppurating Category of Tetanus

2-32 有一患者，腹脹喘促，作渴寒熱，臀腿糜爛，與死肉相
和，如皮囊盛糊。用童便煎四物、桃仁、紅花、柴胡、黃
芩、麥門、花粉，服之頓退。彼用黑羊皮貼之益甚。後砭去
膿血甚多，氣息奄奄，唇口微動，牙關緊急，患處色黯。或
欲用破傷風藥。余曰：此氣血虛而變症也。用參、耆、芎、
歸、白朮，並獨參湯入乳汁，元氣復而諸症愈，及用十全大
補湯，調理而安。

There was a patient with abdominal distension, hasty panting, thirst, and [sensations of] cold and heat. His buttocks and legs were reduced to a pulp [from a beating or caning] that was mixed together with dead flesh like a sack of skin filled with paste. I used child's urine to boil F-8 *Sì Wù Tāng* with *táo rén, hóng huā, chái hú, huáng qín, mài mén dōng*, and *tiān huā fěn*. He took it and the condition immediately receded. He stuck black goat skin on it and the condition increased a lot. Later I *biān*-lanced it and removed quite a lot of pus and blood. He seemed to be breathing his last breaths. His lips and mouth stirred slightly and his jaws were clenched. The affected site was dull-colored. Someone wanted to use herbs for tetanus. I said: This is qì and blood deficiency that has become a transmuted condition. I used *rén shēn, huáng qí, chuān xiōng, dāng guī,* and *bái zhú* along with F-11 *Dú Shēn Tāng* added to milk. His original qì returned and the various conditions recovered. I then used F-16 *Shí Quán Dà Bǔ Tāng*. He took proper care of himself and he was peaceful.

此症若膿瘀內焮者，宜針之 。若潰後口噤遺尿，而類破傷風
等症者，乃氣血虛極也，急用大補之劑 。若素多痰，患風症
者，宜清痰降火 。若因怒而見風症者，宜清肝降火 。若人不
慎房勞，而忽患前症，此由腎水不足，心火熾甚，宜滋陰補
氣血為主 。若誤作風症，治之即死 。

In this condition:

▶ If pus and stasis are scorching inside, it is appropriate to needle [*biān-lance*] it.

▶ If after ulcerating, there is clenched jaw and incontinence of urine, and there is some type of tetanus or similar condition, it is extreme deficiency of qì and blood; quickly use strongly supplementing prescriptions.

▶ If he usually has a lot of phlegm and suffers a wind pattern, use herbs to clear phlegm and descend fire.

▶ If a wind condition appears due to anger, it is appropriate to clear the liver and descend fire.

▶ If a person is incautious with bedroom taxation and suddenly suffers the above condition, this is from insufficiency of kidney water with heart fire strongly blazing; it is appropriate to use yīn enrichment and qì and blood supplemention as the governing principles. If it is mistakenly treated as a wind condition, he will die.

內虛變痙（痓當作痙）

Internal Deficiency Mutating into Tetany

(Chì 痓 should be written as jing 痙[46])

2-33 有一患者，內潰，針出膿三五碗。遂用大補之劑，翌日
熱甚汗出，足冷口噤，腰背反張。眾欲投發散之劑。余曰：
此氣血虛極而變痙也，若認作風治則誤矣。用十全大補等藥
而愈。

There was a patient with internal ulcerations. I needled to take out three or
five bowlfuls of pus. I then used a strongly supplementing prescription. The
next day his fever was high, with sweating, cold feet, clenched jaw, and arched-
back rigidity. Everyone wanted to give him dissipating prescriptions. I said:
This is extreme qì and blood deficiency that has mutated into tetany; treating
it as wind is a mistake. I used F-16 *Shí Quán Dà Bǔ Tāng* and so forth, and he
recovered.

此症多因傷寒汗下過度，與產婦潰瘍氣血虧損所致，但當調
補氣血為善。若服克伐之劑，多致不救。

This condition is often due to excessive use of cold damage prescriptions used
to sweat or descend [promote a bowel movement]. In postpartum women, it
is caused by ulcerating sores and enfeebled qì and blood. Only regulating and
supplementing qì and blood is good. If one takes prescriptions to subdue and
cut down, many will reach the point where they cannot be rescued.

2-34 有一患者，兩月餘矣，瘡口未完，因怒發痙，瘡口出
血。此怒動肝火而為患耳，用柴胡、芩、連、山梔、防風、
桔梗、天麻、鈎藤鈎、甘草，治之頓愈。

---

46. This note correcting a character must have been written by a later editor.

69

The opening of a patient's wound was not completely closed after more than two months. Tetany erupted due to anger and the opening of the wound bled. Anger stirred up liver fire and developed into this form of suffering. I treated him with *chái hú, huáng qín, huáng lián, zhī zǐ, fáng fēng, jié gěng, tiān má, gōu téng gōu,* and *gān cǎo,* and he immediately recovered.

劉宗厚先生云：痙有屬風火之熱內作者，有因七情怒氣而作者，亦有濕熱內盛、痰涎壅遏經絡而作者，惟宜補虛降火，敦土平木，清痰去濕。

Doctor Liú Zōnghòu[47] said: Some types of tetany develop from the heat of wind-fire,[48] some develop from the seven emotions and anger, some also develop from internal abundance of damp-heat and phlegm-drool congesting and obstructing the channels and *luò*-networks; it is only appropriate to supplement deficiency and descend fire, solidify earth and calm wood, clear phlegm and remove dampness.

---

47. Liú Zōnghòu was a doctor who lived at the end of the *Yuán* and the beginning of the *Míng* dynasty. He was a descendant of Liú Wánsù.
48. Some versions of this quotation have 屬風火之熱而作 rather than 屬風火之熱內作. I used this for my translation.

《正體類要・上卷・墜跌金傷治驗》
3. Treatment Experience Regarding Injury from Falls and Tumbles or Wounds from Metal

瘀血腹痛
Blood Stasis with Abdominal Pain

3-1 有一患者，仲秋夜歸墜馬，腹內作痛，飲酒數杯，翌早大便，自下瘀血即安。此元氣充實，挾酒勢而行散也。

In the second month of autumn, a patient fell off his horse while returning home at night. He had pain inside his abdomen and drank several cups of liquor. The next morning during his bowel movement, the blood stasis came out without intervention and then he was peaceful. This was fullness of original qì embracing the power of liquor to move and dissipate blood stasis.

3-2 一男子跌傷，腹痛作渴，食梨子二枚，益甚，大便不通，血欲逆上。用當歸承氣湯加桃仁，瘀血下而瘥。此因元氣不足，瘀血得寒而聚凝也。故產婦金瘡者，不宜食此。

A male was injured by a tumble; he suffered abdominal pain and thirst. He ate two pears and the symptoms increased a lot. He had constipation and his blood was about to counterflow upward.[49] I used F-9a *Dāng Guī Chéng Qì Tāng* adding *táo rén*. The blood stasis descended [with a bowel movement] and he recuperated. This was due to insufficient original qì; blood stasis gathered and congealed after receiving coldness [from the pears]. Thus, it is inappropriate for

---

49. Blood stasis in the abdomen might be let out by descending [promoting a bowel movement] in a strong patient. Here, since the patient ate cold-natured pears, movement slowed down or stopped and so he became constipated. Since the blood stasis could not move down, it might next counterflow up and injure his heart or lungs, or cause vomiting of blood.

women after giving birth or people with wounds inflicted by metal to eat this [cold fruits and the like].

3-3 一男子孟秋墜梯，腹停瘀血。用大黃等藥，其血不下，反加胸膈脹痛，喘促短氣。余用肉桂、木香末各三錢，熱酒調服，即下黑血，及前所服之藥而蘇。此因寒藥凝滯而不行，故用辛溫之劑散之。

During the first month of autumn, a male fell off a ladder. Blood stasis collected in his abdomen. He used herbs like *dà huáng*, but the blood did not descend and contrary to expectations, it added distention and pain of the chest and diaphragm, hasty panting, and shortness of breath. I used three *qián* (11.19 grams) each of powdered *ròu guì* and *mù xiāng* mixed with hot liquor. He took it and then descended black blood along with the previous herbs he had taken. He then revived. This was due to cold herbs that had congealed and stagnated so the stasis did not move; thus using acrid warm prescriptions dissipated it.

脾傷腹痛
Injury to the Spleen with Abdominal Pain

3-4 陳侍御墜馬，腿痛作嘔，服下藥一劑，胸腹脹痛，按之即止，惟倦怠少氣。診其脈，微細而濇。余曰：非瘀血也，乃痛傷氣血，復因藥損脾氣而然耳。投養脾胃、生氣血之藥而愈。

Censor Chén fell off his horse; he had leg pain and vomiting. He took a dose of herbs to descend [promote a bowel movement] and developed distention and pain in his chest and abdomen that stopped when pressed; [his other symptoms were] only fatigue with shortage of qì. I felt his pulse which was faint, fine, and rough. I said: This is not blood stasis; it is this way because pain injured qì and blood, and it is further due to herbs harming spleen qì. I gave him herbs to nourish the spleen and stomach and engender qì and blood. He recovered.

血虛脅脹
Blood Deficiency with Rib-Side Distention

3-5 李進士季夏傷手，出血不止，發熱作渴，兩脅作脹，按之
即止，此血虛也。用八珍加軟柴胡、天花粉，治之頓愈；更
用養氣血之藥，調理而痊。

Metropolitan Graduate Lǐ injured his hand during the last month of summer.
The bleeding would not stop, and he had fever, thirst, and distention of both
rib-sides that stopped when pressed. This was blood deficiency. I treated him
with F-4 *Bā Zhēn Tāng* adding *ruǎn chái hú* and *tiān huā fěn*. He immediately
recovered. I further used herbs to nourish qì and blood. He took proper care of
himself and recuperated.

血虛煩躁
Blood Deficiency with Vexation and Agitation

3-6 吳給事墜馬傷首，出血過多，發熱煩躁，肉瞤筋惕。或欲
投破傷風藥。余曰：此血虛火動所致，當峻補其血為善。遂
用聖愈湯二劑即安，又養氣血而瘡痊。

Supervising Secretary Wú injured his head when he fell off his horse; it was
bleeding excessively, with fever, vexation, agitation, twitching flesh, and jerking
sinews. Someone wanted to give him herbs for tetanus. I said: This is caused by
blood deficiency with fire stirring; drastically supplementing his blood is good.
I then used two doses of F-15 *Shèng Yù Tāng* and he became peaceful. I next
nourished qì and blood and the wound recuperated.

亡血出汗
Collapse of Blood with Sweating

3-7 張進士季秋墜馬，亡血過多，出汗煩躁，翌日其汗自止，熱躁益甚，口噤手顫。此陰血虛，陽火乘之，而汗出為寒氣收斂腠理，故汗不得出，火不得泄，怫鬱內甚，而益增他症也。余用四物加柴胡、黃芩、山梔，四劑少止。又用四物、參、耆、軟柴胡、五味、麥門，治之而痊。

In the last month of autumn, Metropolitan Graduate Zhāng fell off his horse and suffered collapse from excessive bleeding. He was sweating, vexed, and agitated. The next day, the sweating stopped without intervention but the heat and agitation increased a lot. He had clenched jaws and tremors of the hands. This was deficiency of yīn and blood with yáng and fire taking advantage of it; the [lack of] sweating was due to cold qì contracting the *còu lǐ* so he was unable to sweat. The fire could not discharge [with the sweat] and was seriously constrained on the interior, so it increased his symptoms. I used four doses of F-8 *Sì Wù Tāng* adding *chái hú, huáng qín*, and *zhī zǐ*, and the symptoms decreased. I then treated him using F-8 *Sì Wù Tāng* with *rén shēn, huáng qí, ruǎn chái hú, wǔ wèi zǐ*, and *mài mén dōng* and he recuperated.

亡血昏憒（二條）
Dazed from Collapse of Blood (two items)[50]

3-8 一婦人孟冬傷足，亡血頭汗，內熱作渴，短氣煩躁，不時昏憒，其脈洪大，按之微弱。此陰血虛於下，孤陽炎於上，故發厥而頭出汗也。以四物合小柴胡湯一劑，汗即止。以四物去川芎，加參、耆、麥門、五味、炙草，少用肉桂，四劑，諸症悉去。又三十餘劑，血氣復而愈。

---

50. Many headings have more than one item yet they did not all get an enumeration like this. The reason is unknown.

In the first month of winter, a woman injured her foot. She had collapse of blood and was sweating from her head, with internal heat, thirst, shortness of breath, vexation, and agitation. She was frequently in a daze. Her pulse was surging and large but faint and weak when pressed. This was deficiency of yīn and blood in the lower body; solitary yáng flared to the upper body so she had episodes of *jué*-reversal and sweating of the head. I used one dose of F-8 *Sì Wù Tāng* combined with F-2 *Xiǎo Chái Hú Tāng* and the sweating stopped. I used four doses of F-8 *Sì Wù Tāng* removing *chuān xiōng* and adding *rén shēn, huáng qí, mài mén dōng, wǔ wèi zǐ,* and *zhì gān cǎo* with a little *ròu guì*. All conditions were completely removed. I then used more than thirty doses; her blood and qì returned and she recovered.

3-9 一男子孟夏折腿，出血過多，其初眩暈眼花，後則昏憒。此陰血傷損，陽火熾甚，制金不能平木，木旺生風所致。急灌童便，更用人參、當歸各五錢，荊芥、川芎、柴胡、芍藥、白术各二錢，山梔、黃芩、桔梗各一錢，甘草五分，服之隨爽。又用四物、參、耆各三錢，生地、柴胡各一錢，四劑，煩躁悉去。

In the first month of summer, a male broke his leg and bled excessively. In the beginning, he was dizzy with blurry vision. Later he was dazed. This was caused by injury to yīn and blood with yáng fire strongly blazing. The fire restrained metal which was unable to calm wood. Wood was at peak strength and engendered wind. I quickly poured in child's urine and further used five *qián* (18.65 grams) each of *rén shēn* and *dāng guī*; two *qián* (7.46 grams) each of *jīng jiè, chuān xiōng, chái hú, sháo yào,* and *bái zhú*; one *qián* (3.73 grams) each of *zhī zǐ, huáng qín,* and *jié gěng*; and five *fēn* (1.85 grams) of *gān cǎo*. He took it and became lucid. I then used four doses of F-8 *Sì Wù Tāng* with three *qián* (11.19 grams) each of *rén shēn* and *huáng qí*; and one *qián* (3.73 grams) each of *shēng dì* and *chái hú*. The vexation and agitation were completely removed.

濕痰作痛 （三條）
Pain caused by Damp-phlegm (three items)

3-10 大宗伯沈立齋孟冬閃腰作痛，胸間痰氣不利。以枳殼、青皮、柴胡、升麻、木香、茴香、當歸、川芎、赤芍、神曲、紅花，四劑，而瘥。但飲食不甘，微有潮熱。以參、耆、白朮、陳皮、白芍各一錢，歸身二錢，川芎八分，軟柴胡、地骨、炙草各五分，十餘劑而康。

In the first month of winter, Minister of Rites Shěn Lìzhāi painfully wrenched his low back. Phlegm qì within his chest inhibited it. I used four doses of *zhǐ qiào, qīng pí, chái hú, shēng má, mù xiāng, huí xiāng, dāng guī, chuān xiōng, chì sháo, shén qū,* and *hóng huā,* and he recuperated. However, food and drink did not taste sweet and he had a slight tidal fever. I used more than ten doses of: one *qián* (3.73 grams) each of *rén shēn, huáng qí, bái zhú, chén pí,* and *bái sháo;* two *qián* (7.46 grams) of *dāng guī shēn;* eight *fēn* (2.96 grams) of *chuān xiōng;* and five *fēn* (1.85 grams) each of *ruǎn chái hú, dì gǔ pí,* and *zhì gān cǎo,* and he became healthy.

3-11 劉尚寶體肥臀閃作痛，服透骨丹，反致肢節俱痛，下體益甚。以二陳、南星、羌活、防風、牛膝、木瓜、蒼朮、黃芩、黃柏治之，身痛遂安。以前藥加歸尾、赤芍、桔梗，治之而痊。

Liú Shàngbǎo's body was robust but he wrenched his buttocks and had pain. He took UFx-2 *Tòu Gǔ Dān,* but contrary to expectations, it resulted in pain of all the limbs and joints and the pain increased a lot in his lower body. I treated him using UF-3 *Èr Chén Tāng* with *nán xīng, qiāng huó, fáng fēng, niú xī, mù guā, cāng zhú, huáng qín,* and *huáng bǎi.* The generalized pain became peaceful. I treated him using the above herbs adding *dāng guī wěi, chì sháo,* and *jié gěng,* and he recuperated.

3-12 鄭吏部素有濕痰，孟冬墜馬，服辛熱破血之藥，遍身作痛，發熱口乾，脈大而滑，此熱劑激動痰火為患耳。治以清燥湯去人參、當歸、黃耆，加黃芩、山梔、半夏、黃柏，熱痛頓去，患處少愈。用二陳、羌活、桔梗、蒼朮、黃柏、薑製生地、當歸遂痊。

Zhèng from the Ministry of Civil Appointment usually had damp-phlegm. He fell off his horse in the first month of winter and took acrid hot herbs to break blood. His entire body became painful with fever and dry mouth. His pulse was large and slippery. He suffered this due to the use of hot prescriptions that agitated phlegm-fire. I treated him using F-19 *Qīng Zào Tāng*, removing *rén shēn*, *dāng guī*, and *huáng qí* and adding *huáng qín, zhī zǐ, bàn xià*, and *huáng bǎi*. The hot pain was immediately removed and the affected site recovered a little. I use UF-3 *Èr Chén Tāng* with *qiāng huó, jié gěng, cāng zhú, huáng bǎi, shēng dì* that was prepared with ginger, and *dāng guī*. He then recovered.

肝火作痛
Pain caused by Liver Fire

3-13 楊司天，骨已入骹，患處仍痛，服藥不應，肝脈洪大而急。余曰：此肝火盛而作痛也。用小柴胡湯加山梔、黃連，二劑，痛止，用四物、山梔、黃柏、知母，調理而康。

Astronomical Official Yáng [had a dislocation but] the bone had already been reinserted into its socket.[51] The affected site was still painful. He took herbs but did not respond. His liver pulse was surging, large, and urgent. I said: This pain is caused by abundance of liver fire. I used two doses of F-2 *Xiǎo Chái Hú Tāng* adding *zhī zǐ* and *huáng lián*, and the pain stopped. I used F-8 *Sì Wù Tāng* with *zhī zǐ, huáng bǎi*, and *zhī mǔ*. He took proper care of himself and he became healthy.

---

51. One edition of this book has *jiù* 臼 instead of *jiè* 骹. Both can mean the socket of a joint.

血虛作痛
Pain caused by Blood Deficiency

3-14 一婦人磕臂出血，骨痛熱渴，煩悶頭暈，日晡益甚。此陰虛內熱之症，用八珍加丹皮、麥門、五味、骨碎補、肉桂，及地黃丸，治之悉愈；卻去桂，加牛膝、續斷，二十餘劑而瘡愈。

A woman's arm bumped against something and bled, with bone pain, fever, thirst, vexation, oppression, and dizzy head; it increased a lot at sunset. This was a condition of yīn deficiency with internal heat. I treated her using F-4 *Bā Zhēn Tāng* adding *mǔ dān pí, mài mén dōng, wǔ wèi zǐ, gǔ suì bǔ,* and *ròu guì*, as well as F-29 *Dì Huáng Wán*, and she completely recovered. I then gave her more than twenty doses, removing *ròu guì* and adding *niú xī* and *xù duàn*; the wound recovered.

骨傷作痛（二條）
Pain caused by Bone Injury (two items)

3-15 一小兒足傷作痛，肉色不變，傷在骨也。頻用炒蔥熨之，五更用和血定痛丸；日間用健脾胃、生氣血之劑；數日後服地黃丸，三月餘而痊。

A child injured his foot. This caused pain but the color of the flesh did not change; the injury was in the bone. I frequently ironed it with stir-fried *cōng bái* [see F-3 *Cōng Yùn Fǎ*]. During the fifth watch (3 – 5 a.m.) I used F-32 *Hé Xuè Dìng Tòng Wán*. In the daytime I used prescriptions to fortify the spleen and stomach and engender qì and blood. After several days, he took F-29 *Dì Huáng Wán*. He took it for more than three months and recuperated.

3-16 一小兒臂骨出骱接入，腫痛發熱，服流氣等藥益甚，飲
食少思。余以蔥熨之，其痛即止。以六君、黃耆、柴胡、桔
梗、續斷、骨碎補治之，飲食進而腫痛消。又用補中益氣加
麥門、五味治之，氣血和而熱退，愈矣。

A child's humerus came out of its socket and was reinserted. He had swelling, pain, and fever. He took herbs to flow qì and so forth but the symptoms
increased a lot, with little thought of food and drink. I ironed it with *cōng bái*
[see F-3 *Cōng Yùn Fǎ*] and his pain stopped. I treated him using F-34 *Liù Jūn Zǐ
Tāng* with *huáng qí, chái hú, jié gěng, xù duàn*, and *gǔ suì bǔ*. He began to eat and
the swelling and pain dispersed. I then treated him using F-23 *Bǔ Zhōng Yì Qì
Tāng* adding *mài mén dōng* and *wǔ wèi zǐ*. Qì and blood harmonized, the fever
receded, and he recovered.

氣虛血滯
Qì Deficiency with Blood Stagnation

3-17 戴給事墜馬，腿腫痛而色黯，食少倦怠。此元氣虛弱，
不能運散瘀血而然耳，遂用補中益氣去升麻、柴胡，加木
瓜、茯苓、芍藥、白朮，治之而痊。

Supervising Secretary Dài fell off his horse. His leg was swollen, painful, and
dull-colored. His food intake decreased and he felt fatigued. It was this way
because his original qì was deficient and weak so it was unable to transport
blood and dissipate stasis. I then treated him using F-23 *Bǔ Zhōng Yì Qì Tāng*
removing *shēng má* and *chái hú* and adding *mù guā, fú líng, sháo yào*, and *bái zhú*.
He recuperated.

氣虛不潰
Qì Deficiency with Inabilty to Ulcerate

3-18 少宗伯劉五清，臁傷一塊，微痛少食。用六君子湯，倍加當歸、黃耆，其痛漸止，月餘瘀血內涸而不潰，公以為痊。余曰：此陽氣虛極，須調補。不從。至來春，頭暈，痰涎壅塞，服清氣化痰，病勢愈盛，脈洪大而微細。欲以參、耆、歸、朮、附子之類補之。不信。至秋初，因怒昏憒而厥。

Minister Liú Wǔqīng injured his lower leg and had a lump with mild pain and reduced food intake. He used F-34 *Liù Jūn Zǐ Tāng* adding a double dose of *dāng guī* and *huáng qí*. His pain gradually stopped. After more than a month the blood stasis inside dried up and did not ulcerate. The gentleman took this as recovery. I said: This is extreme yáng qì deficiency; we must regulate and supplement. He did not agree. When spring arrived, his head was dizzy and he had phlegm-drool congestion. He took herbs to clear qì and transform phlegm but the force of the disease became more abundant. His pulse was surging and large but faint and fine. I wanted to use herbs like *rén shēn, huáng qí, dāng guī, bái zhú*, and *fù zǐ* to supplement him but he did not have confidence in me. At the beginning of autumn, he was in a daze due to anger and died.

氣虛壅腫（三條）
Qì Deficiency with Obstruction and Swelling (three items)

3-19 一婦人閃臂腕，腫大已三月，手臂日細，肌瘦惡寒，食少短氣，脈息微細。屬形病俱虛也，遂投補中益氣加肉桂，引諸藥以行至臂；再加貝母、香附，以解久病之鬱；間服和血定痛丸，以蔥熨之，腫消二三。因怒，患處仍脹，胸膈兩脅微痛，以前湯更加木香、山梔、半夏、桔梗，服之少可。復因驚，不寐少食，盜汗，以歸脾湯加五味、麥門，二十餘劑，而安，腫消三四，手臂漸肥。但經水過期而少，此

心脾之血尚未充足而然也。乃用八珍加五味、麥門、丹皮、
遠志、香附、貝母、桔梗，四十餘劑，諸症悉愈。後因怒發
熱譫語，經水如涌，此怒動肝火，以小柴胡湯，加生地黃三
錢，一劑遂止。以四物加柴胡，調理而康。

A woman wrenched her wrist and the swelling was still large after three
months. Her arm grew thinner each day and her muscles became emaciated,
with aversion to cold, decreased food intake, and shortness of breath. Her pulse
was faint and fine. This corresponded to deficiency of both the physical body
and qì.[52] I then gave her F-23 *Bǔ Zhōng Yì Qì Tāng* adding *ròu guì* to guide all
the herbs to move through the arm; I also added *bèi mǔ* and *xiāng fù* to resolve
the constraint of enduring disease. She took F-32 *Hé Xuè Dìng Tòng Wán* for
an interval. I ironed the site with *cōng bái* [see F-3 *Cōng Yùn Fǎ*]. The swelling
decreased by twenty or thirty percent. Due to anger, the affected site was still
distended and her chest, diaphragm, and both rib-sides were slightly painful.
I used the previous decoction further adding *mù xiāng, zhī zǐ, bàn xià*, and *jié
gěng*. She took it and got a little better. Again due to fright, she had insomnia,
decreased food intake, and night sweating. I used more than twenty doses of
F-12 *Guī Pí Tāng* adding *wǔ wèi zǐ* and *mài mén dōng* and she was peaceful. The
swelling decreased thirty or forty percent and her arm gradually plumped up.
However, her menstruation was late and reduced in quantity. It was this way because blood of the heart and spleen had not yet filled back up. I then used more
than forty doses of F-4 *Bā Zhēn Tāng* adding *wǔ wèi zǐ, mài mén dōng, mǔ dān pí,
yuǎn zhì, xiāng fù, bèi mǔ*, and *jié gěng*, and all conditions completely recovered.
Later, due to anger, she had fever and delirious speech. Her menstrual fluids
gushed out. This was anger stirring up liver fire. I used one dose of F-2 *Xiǎo
Chái Hú Tāng* adding three *qián* (11.19 grams) of *shēng dì huáng*, and it then
stopped. I used F-8 *Sì Wù Tāng* adding *chái hú*. She took proper care of herself
and became healthy.

---

52. The text has 形病 (disease of the physical body) here but the author uses 形氣
(physical body and qi) in many parallel places of the text. In addition, the use of the
word *both* or *all* (jù 俱) indicates that there should be more than one aspect of deficiency. The translation is based on this.

3-20 州守陳克明子，閃右臂腕，腫痛肉色不變，久服流氣等藥，加寒熱少食，舌乾作渴。余曰：傷損等症，腫不消，色不變，此運氣虛而不能愈，當助脾胃、壯氣血為主。遂從余法治之，不二月形氣漸充，腫熱漸消，半載諸症悉退，體如常。

The son of Regional Guard Chén Kèmíng wrenched his right wrist. It was swollen and painful but the color of the flesh did not change. He took herbs to flow qì and so forth for a long time, but this added [sensations of] cold and heat, decreased food intake, dry tongue, and thirst. I said: If swelling does not disperse and color does not change in injury and related conditions, it is deficiency of transporting qì; this leads to inability to recover. We should assist the spleen and stomach and invigorate qì and blood as the governing principles. Then I treated him following my method. In less than two months, his physical body and qì gradually filled in and the swelling and heat gradually dispersed. In half a year, all the symptoms receded, and his body was back to normal.

3-21 一小兒閃腿腕壅腫，形氣怯弱。余欲治以補氣血為主，佐以行散之劑。不信。乃內服流氣飲，外敷寒涼藥，加寒熱體倦。余曰：惡寒發熱，脈息洪大，氣血虛極也，治之無功。後內潰，瀝盡氣血而亡。

A child wrenched his ankle; it was congested and swollen. His physical body and qì were weak. I wanted to treat him using a prescription with the governing principle of supplementing qì and blood and assist using herbs to move and dissipate, but they did not have confidence in me. They then had him take UFx-3 *Liú Qì Yǐn* internally and applied cold and cooling herbs externally. This added [sensations of] cold and heat and weariness of the body. I said: With aversion to cold, fever, and a surging large pulse, qì and blood are extremely deficient. I treated him without success. Later, it ulcerated internally; a lot of qì and blood trickled out and he died.

瘀血腫痛（二條）

Blood Stasis with Swelling and Pain (two items)

3-22 一男子閃傷右腿，壅腫作痛。余謂：急砭去滯血，以補
元氣，庶無後患。不信。乃外敷大黃等藥，內服流氣飲。後
湧出穢膿數碗許，其膿不止。乃復請治，視其腿細而脈大，
作渴發熱，辭不治，後果歿。

A male had a wrenching injury of his right leg; it was congested, swollen, and
painful. I said: Many people will not suffer later if they quickly receive *biān*-
lancing to remove stagnant blood and also supplement original qì. He did not
have confidence in me. He then applied herbs like *dà huáng* externally and took
UFx-3 *Liú Qì Yǐn* internally. Later, several bowlfuls of foul pus gushed out; the
discharge of pus did not stop. He invited me to treat him again. I saw his leg was
thin but his pulse was large and he had thirst and fever. I took leave of him and
did not treat him,[53] and he consequently died.

3-23 窗友黃汝道，環跳穴處閃傷，瘀血腫痛，發熱作渴。遂
砭去瘀血，知其下焦素有虛火，用八珍加黃柏、知母、牛
膝、骨碎補，四劑頓止。用十全大補湯少加黃柏、知母、麥
門、五味，三十餘劑而斂。

My classmate, Huáng Rǔdào, had a wrenching injury with blood stasis, swelling, and pain at the site of Huán Tiào (GB 30); he was feverish and thirsty. I
then *biān*-lanced it to remove blood stasis. I knew his lower jiāo usually had deficiency fire. I used four doses of F-4 *Bā Zhēn Tāng* adding *huáng bǎi, zhī mǔ, niú
xī,* and *gǔ suì bǔ,* and he immediately recovered. I used more than thirty doses of
F-16 *Shí Quán Dà Bǔ Tāng* adding a little *huáng bǎi, zhī mǔ, mài mén dōng,* and *wǔ
wèi zǐ,* and the wound closed up.

---

53. Xuē did not treat him because he knew the case was hopeless. At the time, doctors
did not intervene in cases when they felt death was inevitable.

筋傷癰腫
Sinew Injury with Obstruction and Swelling

3-24 李考功子十四歲，腳腕閃傷，腫而色夭，日出清膿少許，肝脈微澀。此肝經受傷，氣血虛而不能潰，難治之症也，急止克伐之劑。不信。乃雜用流氣等藥，後果出爛筋而死。

The son of Evaluator Lǐ was fourteen years old. He had a wrenching injury of his ankle with swelling and the region of the injury was a deathly color. It exuded a little clear pus each day. His liver pulse was faint and rough. This was injury to the liver channel with deficiency of qì and blood that resulted in inability to ulcerate. The condition was difficult to treat. I quickly stopped their use of formulas to subdue and cut down. They did not have confidence in me. They then randomly used herbs to flow qì and so forth. Consequently, the sinews putrefied and he died.

肺火衄血
Lung Fire with Spontaneous External Bleeding

3-25 張地官墜馬傷腿，服草烏等藥，致衄血咳嗽，臂痛目黃，口渴齒痛，小便短少。此因燥劑傷肺與大腸而致。余用生地、芩、連、黃柏、知母、山梔、山藥、甘草，以潤肺之燥而生腎水，小便頓長，諸症並止。以山藥、五味、麥門、參、耆、芎、歸、黃柏、黃芩、知母、炙草，以滋陰血、養元氣，而瘡斂。

Minister Zhāng fell off his horse and injured his leg. He took herbs like *căo wū* which resulted in nosebleeds, cough, arm pain, yellow eyes, thirst, toothache, and short scant urination. This was due to drying prescriptions injuring the lungs and large intestine. I used *shēng dì, huáng qín, huáng lián, huáng băi, zhī mŭ, zhī zĭ, shān yào,* and *gān căo* to moisten dryness of the lungs and engender kidney water. His urination immediately lengthened and all conditions simultaneously stopped. I used *shān yào, wǔ wèi zǐ, mài mén dōng, rén shēn, huáng qí, chuān xiōng, dāng guī, huáng bǎi, huáng qín, zhī mǔ,* and *zhì gān cǎo* to enrich yīn and blood and noursh original qì, and the wound closed up.

肝火出血 （三條）
Liver Fire with Bleeding (three items)

3-26 俞進士折腿，骨已接，三月尚發熱，出汗不止，正體醫
治不應。左關脈洪數。此肝火熾甚，血得熱而妄行也。遂投
小柴胡湯加山梔、芍藥、生地、防風，血止熱退。又用八
珍、五味、麥門治之，瘡口即愈。

Metropolitan Graduate Yú broke his leg; the bone was already rejoined [set], but he still had fever with incessant sweating after three months. He did not respond to the treatment of the doctor who repaired his body [the bone setter]. His left *guān* pulse was surging and rapid. This was liver fire blazing intensely; blood received this heat and moved recklessly. I then gave him F-2 *Xiǎo Chái Hú Tāng* adding *zhī zǐ, sháo yào, shēng dì,* and *fáng fēng.* The bleeding stopped and the fever receded. I then treated him using F-4 *Bā Zhēn Tāng* with *wǔ wèi zǐ* and *mài mén dōng.* The opening of the wound then recovered.

3-27 田宗伯侄仲秋因怒跌仆，遍身作痛，發熱衄血，肝脈洪
弦。余曰：久衄脈弦洪，乃肝火盛而制金也。至春則肝木茂
盛而自焚，或戕賊脾土，非易治之症。當滋腎水，以生肝
木，益脾土以生肺金。乃雜用瀉肝火等藥，歿於仲春之月。

In the second month of autumn, the nephew of Minister Tián collapsed and fell due to anger. His entire body was painful, with fever and nosebleeds. His liver pulse was surging and bowstring. I said: Enduring nosebleeds and bowstring[54] surging pulse is abundance of liver fire which restrains metal. When

---

54. The word *bowstring* is absent in some editions.

spring arrives, liver wood will become exuberant and set itself on fire or will thieve from spleen earth; the condition is not easy to treat. We should enrich kidney water to engender liver wood and boost spleen earth to engender lung metal. They then randomly used herbs to drain liver fire and so forth. He died in the second month of spring.

3-28 一婦人因怒仆地，傷面出血，痰盛昏憒，牙關緊急。余曰：此怒動肝火，氣逆怫鬱，神明昏冒，而卒倒也。兩手脈洪大而無倫次。以小柴胡湯加黃連、山梔、芎、歸、橘紅、茯苓、薑汁，治之而蘇。

Due to anger, a woman fell to the ground and injured her face with bleeding. She had abundant phlegm, was dazed, and had clenched jaws. I said: Anger stirred up liver fire so qì counterflowed and was constrained; her spirit-brightness became clouded and veiled. This resulted in sudden collapse. The pulse of both hands was surging and large but without coherence. I treated her using F-2 *Xiǎo Chái Hú Tāng* adding *huáng lián, zhī zǐ, chuān xiōng, dāng guī, jú hóng, fú líng,* and ginger juice, and she revived.

胃 火 作 嘔
Vomiting caused by Stomach Fire

3-29 一膏粱之人，跌腿青腫作痛，服辛熱之藥，反發熱作喘，患處益痛，口乾唇揭。余曰：膏粱之人，內多積熱，夏服辛熱之劑，益其胃火而使然也。頻飲童便，以清胃散加山梔、黃芩治之頓止，患處以蔥熨之，腫即消散。

A well-fed person[55] took a tumble and his leg was *qīng*-green with swelling and pain. He took acrid hot herbs, but contrary to his expectations, he developed fever and panting. The pain increased at the affected site. His mouth was dry and

---

55. *Gāo liáng* 膏粱 (well-fed): This term literally means fatty meats and fine grains. It refers to the diet of someone, usually wealthy, who is quite well-nourished.

his lips were chapped. I said: A well-fed person has a lot of heat accumulating inside; he took acrid hot prescriptions in the summer, increasing his stomach fire and making it this way. I had him drink child's urine frequently and I treated him using F-18 *Qīng Wèi Sǎn* adding *zhī zǐ* and *huáng qín*; it immediately stopped. I ironed the affected site with *cōng bái* [see F-3 *Cōng Yùn Fǎ*] and the swelling dispersed.

陰虛作喘
Panting caused by Yīn Deficiency

3-30 舉人杜克弘墜馬，服下血藥，反作喘，日晡益甚 。此血虛所致耳，非瘀血為患 。遂以四物加參、耆、五味、麥門治之，其喘頓止 。又用補中益氣加五味、麥門而愈 。

Provincial Graduate Dù Kèhóng fell off his horse. He took herbs to descend blood [promote a bowel movement], but contrary to his expectations, he began panting. The symptoms increased a lot at sundown. This was caused by blood deficiency; it was not brought about by blood stasis. I then treated him using F-8 *Sì Wù Tāng* adding *rén shēn, huáng qí, wǔ wèi zǐ,* and *mài mén dōng,* and the panting immediately stopped. I then used F-23 *Bǔ Zhōng Yì Qì Tāng* adding *wǔ wèi zǐ* and *mài mén dōng* and he recovered.

此症果系瘀血蒸熏於肺而喘，只宜活血行血，亦不可下 。若面黑胸脹，或膈痛作喘，當用人參一兩、蘇木二兩，作一劑，水煎急服；緩則不治 。產婦多有此疾 。

If this condition is related to blood stasis steaming and fuming the lungs with panting, it is only appropriate to enliven and move blood; one still cannot descend the blood. If the face is black [dark] with chest distention or there is pain of the diaphragm with panting, one *liǎng* (37.3 grams) of *rén shēn* and two *liǎng* (74.6 grams) of *sū mù* should be used as one dose. Boil it in water and quickly take it. If it is chronic, do not treat it [this way]. Many women have this disease after giving birth.

陰虛發熱
Yīn Deficiency with Fever

3-31 楊進士傷手指，焮痛發熱，服寒涼之藥，致飲食頓減，患處不潰。余用托裏養血之藥，食進瘡潰，後因勞每日晡發熱。此陰虛而內熱也，以四物、軟柴胡、地骨皮乃退、更用養血氣之藥而瘡斂。

Metropolitan Graduate Yáng injured his fingers. He had scorching pain and fever so he took cold and cooling herbs, but it immediately resulted in decreased food and drink intake and the affected site did not ulcerate. I used herbs to draw out the interior and nourish blood. He began eating again and the wound ulcerated. Later, he had fever every day at sunset due to taxation. This was yīn deficiency with internal heat. I used F-8 *Sì Wù Tāng* with *ruǎn chái hú* and *dì gǔ pí* and it receded. I further used herbs to nourish blood and qì, and the wound closed up.

氣血虛熱
Qì and Blood Deficiency with Heat

3-32 一男子墜馬，腹有瘀血。服藥下之，致發熱盜汗、自汗，脈浮澀。余以為重劑過傷氣血所致，投以十全大補湯益甚，時或譫語。此藥力未及而然也。以前藥加炮附子五分，服之即睡，覺來頓安，再劑而痊。

A male fell off his horse and had blood stasis in his abdomen. He took herbs to descend it [promote a bowel movement], but it resulted in fever, night sweating, and spontaneous sweating. His pulse was floating and rough. I took this as caused by excessively heavy prescriptions injuring qì and blood. I gave him F-16 *Shí Quán Dà Bǔ Tāng* but it increased a lot, with delirious speech at times. It was this way because the strength of the medicine had not arrived yet. I used the previous herbs adding five *fēn* (1.85 grams) of *pào fù zǐ*. He took it and then slept. When he awoke, he was immediately peaceful. I gave him another dose and he recuperated.

血不歸經（二條）
Blood Failing to Return to its Channel (two items)

3-33 大尹劉國信金瘡出血，發熱煩躁。屬陰虛為患。用聖愈湯治之，虛火息而血歸經矣。

District Magistrate Liú Guóxìn had a wound inflicted by metal, with bleeding, fever, vexation, and agitation. This corresponded to suffering brought about by yīn deficiency. I treated him using F-15 *Shèng Yù Tāng*. The deficiency fire ceased and blood returned to its channel.[56]

3-34 梁閣老侄金瘡腫痛，出血不止，寒熱口乾。此氣虛血無所附，而血不歸經也。用補中益氣、五味、麥門主之，陽氣復而愈。

The nephew of Grand Secretary Liáng had a wound inflicted by metal with swelling, pain, incessant bleeding, [sensations of] cold and heat, and dry mouth. This was qì deficiency so blood had nothing to enclose it and blood could not return to its channel. I used F-23 *Bǔ Zhōng Yì Qì Tāng* with *wǔ wèi zǐ* and *mài mén dōng* to govern the treatment. Yáng qì returned and he recovered.

氣無所附
Qì Without Anything to Enclose

3-35 舉人余時正金瘡焮痛，出血不止，惡寒發熱。用敗毒等藥愈甚，亡血過多，氣無所附而然耳。遂以黃柏、知母、軟柴胡、玄參、五味、麥門，治之即愈。

Provincial Graduate Yú Shízhèng had a wound inflicted by metal with scorching pain, incessant bleeding, aversion to cold, and fever. He used herbs to conquer toxins and the like but it got more severe. Blood collapsed from excessive bleeding; it was this way because qì had nothing to enclose. I then treated him

---

56. *Blood returned to its channel* implies that the bleeding stopped.

using *huáng bǎi, zhī mǔ, ruǎn chái hú, xuán shēn, wǔ wèi zǐ,* and *mài mén dōng,* and he recovered.

氣血俱虛
Deficiency of Both Qì and Blood

3-36 余北仕時，有留都賈學士子，年十六，患流注已二載，公升北宗伯邀余治。診其脈洪大而數，膿清作渴，食少盜汗，朝寒暮熱。余曰：此氣血俱虛也，先以固氣血為主。午前以四君、芎、歸、炙草；午後以四物、參、耆、麥門、五味，兩月諸症遂可一二。有一醫，用滲和之藥保其必生，治之三月，氣血極虛，而形體骨立。復懇治，余被命南下，後果殁。

When I served as an official in the north, the sixteen-year-old son of Scholar Jiǎ from the old capital had suffered streaming sores[57] for two years already. The gentleman was promoted to Northern Chief Minister [so he was now nearby] and invited me to treat the son. I felt his pulse which was surging, large, and rapid. The pus was clear, and he had thirst, decreased food intake, and night sweating. He was cold in the early morning and hot at sunset. I said: This is deficiency of both qì and blood; first I will use the governing principle of securing qì and blood. Before noon I used F-1 *Sì Jūn Zǐ Tāng* with *chuān xiōng, dāng guī,* and *zhì gān cǎo;* after noon I used F-8 *Sì Wù Tāng, rén shēn, huáng qí, mài mén dōng,* and *wǔ wèi zǐ.* In two months, all conditions had improved ten or twenty percent. There was another doctor who used seeping and harmonizing herbs,[58] guaranteeing that the son would live. He treated the son, but in three months, the son had severe deficiency of qì and blood and his body was skin and bones. They again pleaded with me to treat him, but I was sent south by command. Consequently, the son died.

---

57. Streaming sores are sores in deep layers of the body that make toxins which seem to flow through the flesh.

58. This same case is given in *Wài Kē Shū Yào.* There is says, "seeping and disinhibiting 滲利."

陽氣脫陷
Yáng Desertion and Qì Falling

3-37 梁閣老侄跌傷腿，外敷大黃等藥，內服破血之劑，遂致
內潰。余針出穢膿三碗許，虛証悉具，用大補之劑兩月餘，
少能步履。因勞心，手撒眼閉，汗出如水。或欲用祛風之
劑。余曰：此氣血尚未充足而然也。急以艾炒熱頻熨肚臍並
氣海穴處，以人參四兩、炮附子五錢，煎灌，良久臂少動。
又灌一劑，眼開能言，但氣不能接續。乃以參、耆、歸、朮
四味共一斤，附子五錢水煎，徐徐服之而瘡愈。

The nephew of Grand Secretary Liáng tumbled and injured his leg. Externally he applied herbs like *dà huáng*; internally he took a prescription to break blood. This then resulted in internal ulcerations. I needled to let out about three bowlfuls of foul pus. He had a fully deficient condition so I used strongly supplementing prescriptions for more than two months and he was able to walk a little. Due to taxation of the heart [worry], his hands became limp, his eyes were closed, and he was sweating like water. Someone wanted to use a prescription to dispel wind. I said: It is this way because qì and blood have not yet filled back up. I quickly stir-fried mugwort (*ài*) until it was hot and frequently ironed his umbilicus and the region of Qì Hǎi (Rèn 6). I boiled four *liǎng* (149.2 grams) of *rén shēn* and five *qián* (18.65 grams) of blast-fried *fù zǐ* and poured it in. After a long while his arms moved a little. I then poured in another dose; his eyes opened and he was able to speak. However, qì was unable to reconnect. I then used altogether one *jīn* (596.8 grams) of four herbs: *rén shēn*, *huáng qí*, *dāng guī*, and *bái zhú*, with five *qián* (18.65 grams) of *fù zǐ* boiled in water. He slowly and steadily took it and the wound recovered.

膽經血少
Scant Blood of the Gallbladder Channel

3-38 一女子年十七，閃右臂，微腫作痛，寅申時發熱。余決
其膽經血虛火盛，經水果先期而至。先以四物合小柴胡湯，
四劑，熱退；更以加味四物湯，加香附、地骨皮、山梔各五

分，芩、連、炙草各三分，二十餘劑，其腫亦消；乃去黃
連、山梔，又五十餘劑，經水調而元氣充矣。

A seventeen-year-old girl wrenched her left arm, with slight swelling, pain, and fever during the hours of *yín* (3 – 5 a.m.) and *shēn* (3 – 5 p.m.). I decided that the blood of the gallbladder channel was deficient and there was abundant fire. This resulted in her menstrual period arriving early. I first used four doses of F-8 *Sì Wù Tāng* combined with F-2 *Xiǎo Chái Hú Tāng*, and the fever receded. I further used more than twenty doses of F-8a *Jiā Wèi Sì Wù Tāng*, adding five *fēn* (1.85 grams) each of *xiāng fù, dì gǔ pí,* and *zhī zǐ*; and three *fēn* (1.11 grams) each of *huáng qín, huáng lián,* and *zhì gān cǎo*. The swelling also dispersed. I then removed *huáng lián* and *zhī zǐ*, and gave more than fifty additional doses. Her menstruation became regulated and her original qì filled up.

腎經虛怯（二條）
Kidney Channel Depletion (two items)

3-39 儒者王清之跌腰作痛，用定痛等藥不愈，氣血日衰，面
目黧色。余曰：腰為腎之府，雖曰閃傷，實腎經虛弱所致。
遂用杜仲、補骨脂、五味、山茱、蓯蓉、山藥，空心服；又
以六君、當歸、白朮、神曲各二錢，食遠服。不月而瘥。

Confucian Scholar Wáng Qīngzhī tumbled and had low back pain. He used herbs to settle pain and the like but did not recover. Each day, his qì and blood declined and his face and eyes darkened. I said: The low back is the mansion of the kidneys; even though we say it was wrenched, this really resulted from deficiency and weakness of the kidney channel. I then used *dù zhòng, bǔ gǔ zhī, wǔ wèi zǐ, shān zhū yú, ròu cōng róng,* and *shān yào* to be taken on an empty stomach. I next used F-34 *Liù Jūn Zǐ Tāng* with two *qián* (7.46 grams) each of *dāng guī, bái zhú,* and *shén qū,* to be taken between meals. He recuperated in less then a month.

3-40 一二三歲兒閃腰作痛，服流氣等藥半載不愈。余曰：此
稟腎氣不足，不治之症也。後果歿。

A two or three-year-old child wrenched his low back and it was painful. They gave him herbs to flow qì and so forth for half a year but he did not recover. I said: This is insufficient endowment of kidney qì; a condition that cannot be treated. Consequently, he died.[59]

痛傷胃嘔
Pain Injuring the Stomach with Vomiting

3-41 一婦人傷指，手臂俱腫，微嘔少食，彼以為毒氣內攻。診其脈沉細，此痛傷胃氣所致也。遂刺出膿碗許，先以六君、藿香、當歸而食進，繼以八珍、黃耆、白芷、桔梗，月餘而瘡愈。

A woman injured her finger. Her entire arm became swollen. She vomited a little and decreased her food intake. She took this as toxic qì attacking the interior. I felt her pulse; it was sunken and fine. This was caused by pain injuring stomach qì. I then pricked the site to let out about a bowlful of pus. I first used F-34 *Liù Jūn Zǐ Tāng* with *huò xiāng* and *dāng guī* and she began eating. I followed with F-4 *Bā Zhēn Tāng* plus *huáng qí*, *bái zhǐ*, and *jié gěng*. The wound recovered in more than a month.

氣過肉死（二條）
Qì Obstructed by Dead Flesh (two items)

3-42 一男子修傷足指，色黑不痛而欲脫。余曰：此因陽氣虛，不能運達於患處也，急去之，速服補劑以壯元氣，否則死肉延足，必不救矣。不信。果黑爛上脛而死。

A male injured his toe while tending to it [trimming the nails]; it was black, not painful, and it was about to slough off. I said: This is due to yáng qì deficiency with inability to transport and reach the affected site. Quickly remove it and

---

59. *Insufficient endowment* is another way of saying constitutional deficiency. *Cannot be treated* means there is no chance of recovery.

hurry to take supplementing prescriptions to invigorate original qì; otherwise the dead flesh will extend into the foot and it will be impossible save it. He did not have confidence in me. The result was that the black decay ascended his shin and he died.

大抵手足氣血罕到之地，或生瘡、或傷損，若戕其元氣，邪氣愈盛，潰爛延上必死，不潰而色黯者亦死。若骨斷筋皮尚連者，急剪去之。

Generally speaking, the hands and feet are places where qì and blood can scarcely reach. Maybe sores are engendered or there is an injury, but if you harm the patient's original qì, evil qì becomes more abundant so the festering extends upward and the patient will die. If it does not ulcerate and the color is dull, he will also die. If the bone is severed but the sinews and skin are still connected, quickly amputate it.

3-43 一女年數歲，嚴寒上京，兩足受凍不仁，用湯泡漬，至春十指俱爛，牽連未落。余用托裏之劑，助其陽氣，自潰脫，得保其生。此因寒邪遏絕運氣不至，又加熱湯泡漬，故死而不痛也。

A girl who was several years old traveled to the capital during extremely cold weather. Both feet were exposed to cold and were numb. They soaked her feet in hot water. By spring, all ten toes were completely decayed; they were still connected and did not fall off. I used prescriptions to draw out the interior and assist her yáng qì. The toes ulcerated and sloughed off on their own, guaranteeing that she would live. This was due to the ability of cold evils to completely suppress the transportation of qì so it can not arrive. On top of that, they soaked her feet in hot water, so the flesh died and there was no pain.

余嘗見人之嚴寒而出，凍傷其耳目不知痛，若以手觸之，其耳即落。當以暖處良久，或熱手熨之無恙。若以火烘湯泡，其耳即死，至春必潰脫落矣。北方寒氣損人若此，可不察之！

I have seen people go out in extremely cold weather and get frostbite to the ears and eyes without feeling pain. The ear drops off if you touch it. One should put the person in a warm place for a good long time, or heat the hands by ironing them to make them safe and sound. If fire is used to to warm them or they are soaked in hot water, the ears will die. When spring arrives they ulcerate and drop off. In the north, cold qì harms people like this; isn't this observable?!

涼藥過經 （三條）
Cold Medicine Obstructing the Channels (three items)

3-44 雲間曹於容，為室人中風灌藥，誤咬去指半節，燉痛寒熱。外敷大黃等藥，內服清熱敗毒，患處不痛不潰，膿清寒熱愈甚。余曰：此因涼藥過絕隧道而然也。遂敷玉龍膏以散寒氣，更服六君子湯以壯脾胃。數日後患處微痛，腫處漸消，此陽氣運達患處也。果出稠膿，不數日半指潰脫，更服托裏藥而斂。

Cáo Yúróng was from Yúnjiān.[60] After his wife had wind stroke, he poured in herbs for her. She accidentally bit off half of his finger.[61] He had scorching pain and [sensations of] cold and heat. He applied herbs like *dà huáng* externally; he took prescriptions to clear heat and conquer toxins internally. The affected site was not painful, did not ulcerate, and the pus was clear. The [sensations of] cold and heat got more severe. I said: It is this way because cooling herbs have completely obstructed the tunnels. I then applied F-35 *Yù Lóng Gāo* to dissipate cold qì. He further took F-34 *Liù Jūn Zǐ Tāng* to invigorate the spleen and stomach. Several days later, the affected site was slightly painful and the swelling at the site gradually dispersed. This was yáng qì transporting and reaching the affected site. The result was that thick pus exuded and the [injured] half of the finger ulcerated and was sloughed off in just a few days. He further took herbs to draw out the interior and the wound closed up.

---

60. Yúnjiān is another name for Sōngjiāng 松江, now a part of suburban Shànghǎi.
61. The finger must have still been semi-attached for the rest of the case to make sense.

3-45 上舍王天爵，傷足㾴腫，內熱作渴，內服外敷，皆寒涼
敗毒，患處益腫而不潰，且惡寒少食，欲作嘔吐。余曰：此
氣血俱虛，又因寒藥凝結隧道，損傷胃氣，以致前症耳。遂
用香砂六君子、芎、歸、炮薑，外症悉退；惟體倦晡熱，飲
食不甘，以補中益氣湯加地骨皮、五味、麥門，治之而愈。

National University student Wàng Tiānjué injured his foot. He had scorching
swelling, internal heat, and thirst. Internally he took and externally he applied all
cold and cooling herbs to conquer toxins. The swelling increased at the affected
site but it did not ulcerate. Furthermore, he developed aversion to cold, decreased his food intake, and was nauseated. I said: This condition has resulted
from deficiency of both qì and blood and is also due to cold herbs congealing
the tunnels and injuring stomach qì. I then used F-34a *Xiāng Shā Liù Jūn Zǐ
Tāng* with *chuān xiōng*, *dāng guī*, and *pào jiāng*. The whole external condition
receded. The only remaining symptoms were weariness of the body, late afternoon fever, and food and drink did not taste sweet. I treated him using F-23 *Bǔ
Zhōng Yì Qì Tāng* adding *dì gǔ pí*, *wǔ wèi zǐ*, and *mài mén dōng*, and he recovered.

3-46 州守王廷用傷指，即用帛裹之，瘀血內潰，㾴腫至手。
余謂：宜解患處，以出瘀血，更用推陳致新之劑。不信。乃
敷涼藥，痛雖少止，次日復作。又敷之，數日後手心背俱潰
出瘀穢膿水，尚服敗毒之劑，氣血益虛，色黯膿清，飲食少
思，仍請余治，投以壯脾胃、生氣血之劑，由是膿水漸稠而
愈。

Regional Guard Wáng Tíngyòng injured his finger and then bound it with silk.
Blood stasis ulcerated internally and the scorching swelling reached into his
hand. I said: It is appropriate to unwrap the affected site, to let the blood stasis
out, and to further use prescriptions to remove the old and invite the new. He
did not have confidence in me. He then applied cooling herbs. Although the
pain decreased, the next day it returned. He reapplied them. Several days later
both the palm and the back of his hand had ulcerated and discharged static
blood and foul pus-water. He continued to take prescriptions to conquer toxins. The deficiency of qì and blood increased; the color of the wound was dull
and the pus was clear. He had little thought of food and drink. He again invited

me to treat him. I gave him a prescription to invigorate the spleen and stomach and engender qì and blood. From this, the pus-water gradually thickened and he recovered.

《正體類要‧上卷‧湯火所傷治驗》
4. Treatment Experience Regarding Scalds and Burns

火毒刑肺金
Fire Toxins Punishing Lung Metal

4-1 一男子孟冬火傷臂作痛，喘嗽發熱。此火毒刑肺金之症，用人參平肺散治之，喘嗽乃止。因勞又惡寒發熱，此氣血虛也，以八珍湯加桔梗、白芷，治之而退。再加薄桂三分以助藥熱、溫氣血，壞肉潰之而愈。

During the first month of winter, a male received a painful burn on his arm. He also had panting, cough, and fever. This was a condition of fire toxins punishing lung metal. I treated him with F-27 *Rén Shēn Píng Fèi Sǎn* and the panting and cough stopped. Due to taxation he again suffered aversion to cold and fever. This was qì and blood deficiency. I treated him with F-4 *Bā Zhēn Tāng* adding *jié gěng* and *bái zhǐ*, and the symptoms receded. I also added three *fēn* (1.11 grams) of *báo guì* [another name for *ròu guì*] to assist the herbal heat and warm qì and blood. The disintegrated flesh ulcerated and he recovered.

若初起焮赤作痛，用神效當歸膏敷之，輕者自愈，重者自腐，生肌神效。或用側柏葉末，蠟油調敷亦效。若發熱作渴，小便赤色，其脈洪數而實者，用四物、茯苓、木通、生甘草、炒黃連。脈雖洪數而虛者，用八珍。若患處不潰而色黯者，四君、芎、歸、黃耆之類。若肉死已潰而不生肌者，用四君、黃耆、當歸、炮薑。若愈後而惡寒，陽氣未復也，急用十全大補。切不可用寒涼，反傷脾胃。

► If a recent wound is scorching, red, and painful, apply F-41 *Shén Xiào Dāng Guī Gāo* to it. If it is a mild case, he will automatically recover; if serious, it will automatically putrefy and grow muscle. It is divinely effective.

◊ Or it is also effective to apply *cè bǎi yè* powder mixed with beeswax and oil.[62]

▶ If there is fever, thirst, and red urine, with a surging, rapid, and excess pulse, use F-8 *Sì Wù Tāng* with *fú líng, mù tōng, shēng gān cǎo*, and stir-fried *huáng lián*.

  ◊ However, if the pulse is surging, rapid, and deficient, use F-4 *Bā Zhēn Tāng*.

▶ If the affected site does not ulcerate and the color is dull, use herbs like F-1 *Sì Jūn Zǐ Tāng* with *chuān xiōng, dāng guī*, and *huáng qí*.

▶ If the dead flesh has already ulcerated but it does not grow new muscle, use F-1 *Sì Jūn Zǐ Tāng* with *huáng qí, dāng guī*, and *pào jiāng*.

▶ If there is aversion to cold after recovery, yáng qì has not yet returned; quickly use F-16 *Shí Quán Dà Bǔ Tāng*. Be sure not to use cold and cooling herbs, or contrary to expectations, the spleen and stomach will be injured.

火毒燋作
Scorching Fire Toxins

4-2 一男子因醉被湯傷腿，潰爛發熱，作渴飲水，脈洪數而有力。此火毒為患，用生地、當歸、芩、連、木通、葛根、甘草，十餘劑諸症漸退；卻用參、耆、白朮、芎、歸、炙草、芍藥、白芷、木瓜，新肉將完。因勞忽寒熱，此氣血虛而然也，仍用參、耆之藥加五味子、酸棗仁而安；又月餘而瘡痊。

A male scalded his leg when he was drunk. It festered and he had fever, thirst, and he drank water. His pulse was surging, rapid, and forceless. Fire toxins had brought about this disaster. I used more than ten doses of *shēng dì, dāng guī, huáng qín, huáng lián, mù tōng, gé gēn,* and *gān cǎo*. All conditions gradually receded. From then on I used *rén shēn, huáng qí, bái zhú, chuān xiōng, dāng guī, zhì gān cǎo, sháo yào, bái zhǐ,* and *mù guā*. When the new flesh was about to be complete, he suddenly had [sensations of] cold and heat due to taxation. It was this way because of deficiency of qì and blood. I continued to use the *rén shēn*

---

62. One would melt some beeswax into hot oil (perhaps sesame oil) then stir in the *cè bǎi yè* powder and let it cool.

and *huáng qí* formula adding *wǔ wèi zǐ* and *suān zǎo rén* and he was peaceful. The wound recovered after more than a month.

火毒行於下焦
Fire Toxins Traveling to the Lower Jiāo

4-3 一男子火傷兩臂燉痛，大小便不利。此火毒傳於下焦，用生地黄、當歸、芍藥、黄連、木通、山梔、赤茯苓、甘草，一劑，二便清利，其痛亦止。乃以四物、參、耆、白芷、甘草，而壞肉去，又數劑而新肉生。

A male had burns on both arms with scorching pain and inhibited urination and defecation. This was fire toxins being transmitted to the lower jiāo. I used one dose of *shēng dì huáng, dāng guī, sháo yào, huáng lián, mù tōng, zhī zǐ, chì fú líng,* and *gān cǎo*. His elimination became peaceful and his pain also stopped. I then used F-8 *Sì Wù Tāng* with *rén shēn, huáng qí, bái zhǐ,* and *gān cǎo,* and the disintegrated flesh was gone. New flesh grew after several more doses.

火毒乘血分
Fire Toxins Taking Advantage of the Blood Division

4-4 一婦人湯傷胸大潰，兩月不斂，脈洪大而無力，口乾發熱，日晡益甚。此陰血虛火，毒乘之而為患耳。用四物湯加柴胡、丹皮，熱退身涼。更用逍遙散加陳皮，以養陰血、壯脾胃，腐肉去而新肉生。

A woman was scalded on her chest. There were large ulcerations that did not close for two months. Her pulse was surging and large but forceless. She had dry mouth and fever that increased a lot at sunset. This was yīn and blood deficiency fire; toxins took advantage of it and brought about this disaster. I used F-8 *Sì Wù Tāng* adding *chái hú* and *mǔ dān pí*. The fever receded and her body became cool. I further used UF-8 *Xiāo Yáo Sǎn* adding *chén pí* to nourish yīn and blood and invigorate the spleen and stomach; the putrid flesh was gone and new flesh grew.

Volume 2

《正體類要・下卷・方藥》
5. Herbal Formulas

F-1 Sì Jūn Zǐ Tāng 四君子湯
Four Gentlemen Decoction

治脾胃虛弱，或因克伐，腫痛不散，或潰而不斂，或飲食少思，或欲作嘔，大便不實等症。

Treats deficiency and weakness of the spleen and stomach due to [inappropriate use of formulas to] subdue and cut down when swelling and pain do not dissipate; or ulcerations do not close up; or there is little thought of food and drink; or a desire to retch with unformed stool, and similar conditions.

人參白朮茯苓（各二錢）甘草（炙，一錢）

rén shēn	人參		two qián	7.46 g
bái zhú	白朮		two qián	7.46 g
fú líng	茯苓		two qián	7.46 g
gān cǎo	甘草	mix-fried	one qián	3.73 g

上作一劑，薑棗水煎服。

The above makes one dose. Boil in water with ginger and *zǎo*-dates and take it.

F-2 Xiǎo Chái Hú Tāng 小柴胡湯
Minor Chái Hú Decoction

治一切撲傷等症，因肝膽經火盛作痛，出血自汗，寒熱往
來，日晡發熱，或潮熱身熱，咳嗽發熱，脅下作痛，兩肱痞
滿。

Treats all types of injuries from beatings and similar conditions when there is
pain, bleeding, spontaneous sweating, alternating chills and fever, and fever at
sunset; or tidal fever with generalized heat, cough, fever, pain below the rib-
sides, and *pǐ*-glomus with fullness of both flanks due to abundance of fire in the
liver and gallbladder channels.

柴胡（二錢）黃芩（一錢五分）半夏（一錢）人參（一錢）
甘草（炙，三分）

chái hú	柴胡		two qián	7.46 g
huáng qín	黃芩		1.5 qián	5.6 g
bàn xià	半夏		one qián	3.73 g
rén shēn	人參		one qián	3.73 g
gān cǎo	甘草	mix-fried	three fēn	1.11 g

上薑水煎服。

Boil the above in water with ginger and take it.

F-3 Shén Xiào Cōng Yùn Fǎ 神效蔥熨法
Wondrously Effective Ironing Method with Scallions

治跌撲傷損。

Treats injuries from tumbles and beatings.

用蔥白細切杵爛，炒熱敷患處，如冷易之 。腫痛即止，其效
如神 。

Pestle thinly sliced *cōng bái* to a pulp, stir-fry until hot, and apply it to the affected site. Change it when it gets cold. Swelling and pain will stop. Its effects are wondrous.

F-4 Bā Zhēn Tāng 八珍湯
Eight Gem Decoction

治傷損等症，失血過多，或因克伐，血氣耗損，惡寒發熱，
煩躁作渴等症 。

Treats injuries and similar conditions when there is excessive loss of blood; or consumption of blood and qì due to [inappropriate use of formulas to] subdue and cut down, with aversion to cold, fever, vexation, agitation, thirst, and similar conditions.

人參白朮白茯苓當歸川芎白芍藥熟地黃（ 各一錢 ）甘草
（ 炙，五分 ）

rén shēn	人參		one qián	3.73 g
bái zhú	白朮		one qián	3.73 g
bái fú líng	白茯苓		one qián	3.73 g
dāng guī	當歸		one qián	3.73 g
chuān xiōng	川芎		one qián	3.73 g
bái sháo yào	白芍藥		one qián	3.73 g
shú dì huáng	熟地黃		one qián	3.73 g
gān cǎo	甘草	mix-fried	five fēn	1.85 g

上薑棗水煎服 。

Boil the above in water with ginger and *zǎo*-dates and take it.

F-5 Xī Jiǎo Dì Huáng Tāng 犀角地黃湯
Xī Jiǎo and Dì Huáng Decoction[63]

治火盛，血熱妄行，或吐衄不止，大便下血。如因怒而致，加山梔、柴胡。

Treats abundance of fire and blood heat with reckless movement, perhaps spitting blood incessantly, external bleeding [such as nosebleeds], or blood in the stool. If it is caused by anger, add *zhī zǐ* and *chái hú*.

犀角（鎊末）生地黃白芍藥黃芩牡丹皮黃連（各一錢五分）

xī jiǎo	犀角	file into powder	1.5 qián	5.6 g
shēng dì huáng	生地黃		1.5 qián	5.6 g
bái sháo yào	白芍藥		1.5 qián	5.6 g
huáng qín	黃芩		1.5 qián	5.6 g
mǔ dān pí	牡丹皮		1.5 qián	5.6 g
huáng lián	黃連		1.5 qián	5.6 g

用水煎熟，傾於盅內，入犀末服之。

Boil [all the herbs except *xī jiǎo*] in water until cooked, pour it into a cup, add the *xī jiǎo* powder, and take it.

F-6 Shí Wèi Shēn Sū Yǐn 十味參蘇飲
Ten Ingredient Rén Shēn and Zǐ Sū Drink

治氣逆，血蘊上焦，發熱氣促，或咳血衄血，或痰嗽不止。

Treats qì counterflow when blood amasses in the upper jiāo, with fever and hasty breathing; or coughing up blood and external bleeding [such as nosebleeds]; or incessant cough with phlegm.

人參紫蘇半夏茯苓陳皮桔梗前胡葛根枳殼（各一錢）甘草（炙，五分）

---

63. This formula cannot be used today as *xī jiǎo* comes from an endangered species.

rén shēn	人參		one qián	3.73 g
zǐ sū	紫蘇		one qián	3.73 g
bàn xià	半夏		one qián	3.73 g
fú líng	茯苓		one qián	3.73 g
chén pí	陳皮		one qián	3.73 g
jié gěng	桔梗		one qián	3.73 g
qián hú	前胡		one qián	3.73 g
gé gēn	葛根		one qián	3.73 g
zhǐ qiào	枳殼		one qián	3.73 g
gān cǎo	甘草	mix-fried	five fēn	1.85 g

加黃芩、山梔，即加味參蘇飲 。

Adding *huáng qín* and *zhī zǐ* makes it F-6a *Jiā Wèi Shēn Sū Yǐn* (Supplemented Rén Shēn and Zǐ Sū Drink).

上用薑水煎服 。

Boil the above in water with ginger and take it.

F-7 Èr Wèi Shēn Sū Yǐn 二味參蘇飲
Two Ingredient Rén Shēn and Sū Mù Drink

治出血過多，瘀血入肺，面黑喘促 。

Treats bleeding excessively when blood stasis enters the lungs, with black [dark] face and hasty panting.

人參（ 一兩 ）蘇木（ 二兩 ）

rén shēn	人參	one liǎng	37.3 g
sū mù	蘇木	two liǎng	74.6 g

用水煎服 。

Boil in water and take it.

F-8 Sì Wù Tāng 四物湯
Four Agents Decoction

治一切血虛，日晡發熱，煩躁不安者，皆宜服之 。

Treats all types of blood deficiency with fevers at sunset, vexation, agitation, and disquiet. It is appropriate to take for all these symptoms.

當歸熟地黃（ 各三錢 ）芍藥（ 二錢 ）川芎（ 一錢五分 ）

dāng guī	當歸	three qián	11.19 g
shú dì huáng	熟地黃	three qián	11.19 g
sháo yào	芍藥	two qián	7.46 g
chuān xiōng	川芎	1.5 qián	5.6 g

上水煎服 。

Boil the above in water and take it.

加白朮 、茯苓 、柴胡 、丹皮，即加味四物湯 。

Adding *bái zhú, fú líng, chái hú,* and *mǔ dān pí* makes it F-8a *Jiā Wèi Sì Wù Tāng* (Supplemented Four Agents Decoction).

F-9 Táo Rén Chéng Qì Tāng 桃仁承氣湯
Táo Rén Qì-Coordinating Decoction

加當歸即歸承湯 。

Adding *dāng guī* makes it F-9a *Guī Chéng Tāng* (Dāng Guī Coordinating Decoction).

治傷損血滯於內作痛，或發熱發狂等症 。

Treats injury when there is blood stagnation on the interior that leads to pain, or fever with mania and similar conditions.

桃仁芒硝甘草（ 各一錢 ）大黃（ 二錢 ）

táo rén	桃仁	one qián	3.73 g
máng xiāo	芒硝	one qián	3.73 g
gān cǎo	甘草	one qián	3.73 g
dà huáng	大黃	two qián	7.46 g

用水煎服 。大黃更量虛實 。

Boil in water and take it. Adjust the amount of *dà huáng* based on the patient's deficiency or excess.

F-10 Jiā Wèi Chéng Qì Tāng 加味承氣湯
Supplemented Qì-Coordinating Decoction

治瘀血內停，胸腹脹痛，或大便不通等症 。

Treats blood stasis collecting on the interior with chest and abdominal distention and pain, or constipation and similar conditions.

大黃朴硝（ 各二錢 ）枳實（ 一錢 ）厚朴（ 一錢 ）甘草（ 五分 ）當歸紅花（ 各一錢 ）

dà huáng	大黃	two qián	7.46 g
pò xiāo	朴硝	two qián	7.46 g
zhǐ shí	枳實	one qián	3.73 g
hòu pǔ	厚朴	one qián	3.73 g
gān cǎo	甘草	five fēn	1.85 g
dāng guī	當歸	one qián	3.73 g
hóng huā	紅花	one qián	3.73 g

用酒水各一鐘，煎一鐘服 。仍量虛實加減，病急不用甘草 。

Boil in one cup each of liquor and water; boil it down to one cup and take it. As in the previous formula, adjust the amounts based on the patient's deficiency or excess. If the disease is acute, do not use *gān cǎo*.

F-11 Dú Shēn Tāng 獨參湯
Pure Rén Shēn Decoction

治一切失血，與瘡瘍潰後，氣血俱虛，惡寒發熱，作渴煩躁者，宜用此藥補氣。蓋血生於氣，陽生陰長之理也。

Treats all types of blood loss with sores or wounds after ulceration when there is deficiency of both qì and blood, with aversion to cold, fever, thirst, vexation, and agitation: it is appropriate to use this medicine to supplement qì. This must be [used for blood loss] because blood is engendered by qì; this is the theory that "yáng engenders and yīn grows."[64]

用人參二兩，棗十枚，水煎服。

Boil two *liǎng* (74.6 grams) of *rén shēn* with ten *zǎo*-dates in water and take it.

F-12 Guī Pí Tāng 歸脾湯
Spleen-Returning Decoction

治跌撲等症，氣血損傷，或思慮傷脾，血虛火動，寤而不寐，或心脾作痛，怠惰嗜臥，怔忡驚悸，自汗盜汗，大便不調，或血上下妄行，其功甚捷。

Treats injuries from tumbles, beatings, and similar conditions when qì and blood are injured; or thought and contemplation injure the spleen and there is blood deficiency with fire stirring; the patient is awake and cannot sleep; or there is heart and spleen pain, fatigue, somnolence, palpitations, fright palpitations, spontaneous sweating, night sweating, and stool irregulatities; or blood moves recklessly upward and downward. Its results are very quick.

---

64. The statement that "陽生陰長 yáng engenders and yīn grows" comes from *Sù Wèn • Yīn Yáng Yīng Xiàng Dà Lùn*《素問·陰陽應象大論篇第五》, Chapter 5 and *Sù Wèn • Tiān Yuán Jì Dà Lùn*《素問·天元紀大論篇第六十六》, Chapter 66.

白朮當歸白茯苓黃耆（炒）龍眼肉遠志酸棗仁（炒，各一
錢）木香（五分）甘草（炙，三分）人參（一錢）

bái zhú	白朮		one qián	3.73 g
dāng guī	當歸		one qián	3.73 g
bái fú líng	白茯苓		one qián	3.73 g
huáng qí	黃耆	stir-fry	one qián	3.73 g
lóng yǎn ròu	龍眼肉		one qián	3.73 g
yuǎn zhì	遠志		one qián	3.73 g
suān zǎo rén	酸棗仁	stir-fry	one qián	3.73 g
mù xiāng	木香		five fēn	1.85 g
gān cǎo	甘草	mix-fried	three fēn	1.11 g
rén shēn	人參		one qián	3.73 g

上薑棗水煎服。

Boil the above in water with ginger and *zǎo*-dates and take it.

加柴胡、山梔，即加味歸脾湯。

Adding *chái hú* and *zhī zǐ* makes it F-12a *Jiā Wèi Guī Pí Tāng* (Supplemented Spleen-Returning Decoction).

F-13 Rùn Cháng Wán 潤腸丸
Intestine-Moistening Pill

治跌撲等症，或脾胃伏火，大腸乾燥，或風熱血結等症。

Treats injuries from tumbles, beatings, and similar conditions; or deep-lying fire of the spleen and stomach with large intestine dryness; or bound blood due to wind-heat and similar conditions.

麻子仁（一兩）桃仁（一兩，去皮尖）羌活當歸尾大黃
（煨）皂角刺秦艽（各五錢）

110

má zǐ rén	麻子仁		one liǎng	37.3 g
táo rén	桃仁	remove the skin and tips	one liǎng	37.3 g
qiāng huó	羌活		five qián	18.65 g
dāng guī wěi	當歸尾		five qián	18.65 g
dà huáng	大黃	roasted	five qián	18.65 g
zào jiǎo cì	皂角刺		five qián	18.65 g
qín jiāo	秦艽		five qián	18.65 g

上為末，煉蜜丸，桐子大，豬膽汁丸尤妙。每服三五十丸，
食前白滾湯送下。

Powder the above. Make it into pills the size of *wú tóng zǐ* (about 0.6-0.9 centimeters in diameter) with processed honey; making pills with pig bile is especially wonderful. Each dose is thirty to fifty pills taken before meals and swallowed with plain boiled water.

凡怯弱人，先用豬膽導之，不通，宜補氣血。

Whenever the patient is physically weak, first use pig bile as an enema; if that doesn't free the stool, use herbs to supplement qì and blood.

F-14 Dāng Guī Bǔ Xuè Tāng 當歸補血湯
Dāng Guī Blood-Supplementing Decoction

治杖瘡金瘡等症，血氣損傷，肌熱大渴引飲，目赤面紅，晝
夜不息，其脈洪大而虛，重按全無。此病多得於飢渴勞役
者，若誤用白虎湯，必死。

Treats wounds from caning, wounds inflicted by metal, and similar conditions when there is injury to blood and qì, with hot muscles, great thirst with desire to drink, red eyes and face, and this is ceaseless day and night. The pulse is surging and large but deficient; it feels like nothing is there when pressed heavily. In many, this disease is obtained through hunger and thirst or forced labor; if one mistakenly uses UFx-4 *Bái Hǔ Tāng*, the patient will die.

111

黃耆（ 炙，一兩 ）當歸（ 二錢，酒製 ）

| huáng qí | 黃耆 | mix-fried | one liǎng | 37.3 g |
| dāng guī | 當歸 | prepared with liquor | two qián | 7.46 g |

用水煎服 。

Boil in water and take it.

F-15 Shèng Yù Tāng 聖愈湯
Sagacious Cure Decoction

治杖瘡、金瘡、癰疽，膿血出多，熱躁不安，或晡熱作渴等
症 。

Treats wounds from caning, wounds inflicted by metal, or abscesses when
they exude a lot of pus and blood, with heat agitation and lack of peace; or late
afternoon fever with thirst and similar conditions.

熟地黃（ 酒洗 ）生地黃（ 酒洗 ）人參（ 各一錢 ）川芎（ 一
錢 ）當歸（ 酒洗 ）黃芩（ 各五分 ）

shú dì huáng	熟地黃	washed in liquor	one qián	3.73 g
shēng dì huáng	生地黃	washed in liquor	one qián	3.73 g
rén shēn	人參		one qián	3.73 g
chuān xiōng	川芎		one qián	3.73 g
dāng guī	當歸	washed in liquor	five fēn	1.85 g
huáng qín	黃芩		five fēn	1.85 g

用水煎服 。

Boil in water and take it.

F-16 Shí Quán Dà Bǔ Tāng 十全大補湯
Perfect Major Supplementation Decoction

治杖瘡，氣血俱虛，腫痛不消，腐而不潰，潰而不斂，或惡
寒發熱，自汗盜汗，飲食少思，肢體倦怠。若怯弱之人，患
處青腫而肉不壞者，服之自愈。若有瘀血，砭刺早者，服之
自消。或潰而膿水清稀，肌肉不生，或口乾作渴而飲湯者，
尤宜服之。

Treats wounds from caning when there is deficiency of both qì and blood, with
swelling and pain that does not disperse, putrefication without ulceration[65] or it
ulcerates but does not close up; or there is aversion to cold, fever, spontaneous
sweating, night sweating, little thought of food and drink, and fatigued body.
If the patient is weak, the affected site will be *qīng*-green, swollen, and the flesh
will not disintegrate. He will automatically recover when he takes this formula.
If there is blood stasis because the affected site was pricked with a *biān*-lance
too early, the swelling and pain will automatically disperse when he takes this.
Perhaps it has ulcerated with clear thin pus-water and the muscles and flesh do
not grow back; or there is dry mouth and thirst but he drinks hot water – it is
especially appropriate to take this in these cases.

白茯苓人參當歸白朮黃耆川芎白芍藥（炒）熟地黃（生者自
製）肉桂（五分）甘草（炙，各一錢）

bái fú líng	白茯苓		one qián	3.73 g
rén shēn	人參		one qián	3.73 g
dāng guī	當歸		one qián	3.73 g
bái zhú	白朮		one qián	3.73 g
huáng qí	黃耆		one qián	3.73 g
chuān xiōng	川芎		one qián	3.73 g
bái sháo yào	白芍藥	stir-fry	one qián	3.73 g
shú dì huáng	熟地黃	prepare it from the fresh yourself	one qián	3.73 g
ròu guì	肉桂		five fēn	1.85 g
gān cǎo	甘草	mix-fried	one qián	3.73 g

65. In other words, the affected site putrefies under the skin, but since the wound has
not opened up, toxns are retained inside the body.

用薑棗水煎服 。

Boil in water with ginger and *zǎo*-dates and take it.

F-17 Shēn Fù Tāng 參 附 湯
Rén Shēn and Fù Zǐ Decoction

治金瘡 、杖瘡，失血過多，或膿瘀大泄，陽隨陰走，上氣喘
急，自汗盜汗，氣短頭暈等症 。

Treats wounds inflicted by metal or wounds from caning when there is excessive loss of blood or great discharge of pus and static blood. Yáng follows when yīn escapes, so there is ascent of qì, rapid panting, spontaneous sweating, night sweating, shortness of breath, dizzy head, and similar conditions.

人參（ 四錢 ）附子（ 炮去皮臍，三錢 ）

rén shēn	人參		four qián	14.92 g
fù zǐ	附子	blast-fry, remove the skin and 'umbilicus'	three qián	11.19 g

用水煎服 。陽氣脫陷者，倍用之 。

Boil in water and take it. If there is yáng desertion and qì falling, double the dose.

F-18 Qīng Wèi Sǎn 清 胃 散
Stomach-Clearing Powder

治血傷火盛，或胃經濕熱，唇口腫痛，牙齦潰爛，或發熱惡
寒等症 。

Treats injury to blood with fire abundance; or damp-heat of the stomach channel with swelling and pain of the lips and mouth and festering teeth and gums; or fever and aversion to cold and similar conditions.

生地黄（ 五分 ）升麻（ 一錢 ）牡丹皮（ 五分 ）當歸（ 酒洗，
五分 ）黃連（ 五分 ）

shēng dì huáng	生地黄		five fēn	1.85 g
shēng má	升麻		one qián	3.73 g
mǔ dān pí	牡丹皮		five fēn	1.85 g
dāng guī	當歸	washed in liquor	five fēn	1.85 g
huáng lián	黃連		five fēn	1.85 g

用水煎服。如痛未止，黃芩、石膏、大黃之類，皆可量加。

Boil in water and take it. If the pain doesn't stop, herbs like *huáng qín, shí gāo,* or *dà huáng* can be added in.

F-19 Qīng Zào Tāng 清燥湯
Dryness-Clearing Decoction

治跌撲瘡瘍，血氣損傷，或潰後氣血虛怯，濕熱乘之，遍身
酸軟；或秋夏濕熱太甚，肺金受傷，絕寒水生化之源，腎無
所養，小便赤澀，大便不調；或腰腿痿軟，口乾作渴，體重
麻木；或頭目暈眩，飲食少思；或自汗體倦，胸滿氣促；或
氣高而喘，身熱而煩。

Treats injuries from tumbles and beatings, or wounds with injury to blood and qì; or damp-heat taking advantage of qì and blood depletion after ulceration so the entire body is sore and weak; or lung metal injured by extreme damp-heat of autumn and summer. This cuts off the source of engenderment and transformation for cold water[66] so the kidneys have nothing to nourish them, with rough red urination and stool irregularities; or *wěi*-wilting and limpness of the low back and legs with dry mouth, thirst, and heavy numb body; or dizzy head and eyes with little thought of food and drink; or spontaneous sweating, weary body, chest fullness, and hasty breathing; or shallow breathing and panting, generalized heat, and vexation.

---

66. This means that metal cannot engender the kidneys, which correspond to coldness and water.

黃耆（ 一錢五分 ）蒼朮（ 一錢 ）白朮陳皮澤瀉（ 各五分 ）五
味子（ 九粒 ）白茯苓人參升麻（ 各五分 ）麥門冬當歸身生地
黃神曲（ 炒 ）豬苓酒柏（ 各五分 ）柴胡黃連甘草（ 炙，各三
分 ）

huáng qí	黃耆		1.5 qián	5.6 g
cāng zhú	蒼朮		one qián	3.73 g
bái zhú	白朮		five fēn	1.85 g
chén pí	陳皮		five fēn	1.85 g
zé xiè	澤瀉		five fēn	1.85 g
wǔ wèi zǐ	五味子		nine pieces	
bái fú líng	白茯苓		five fēn	1.85 g
rén shēn	人參		five fēn	1.85 g
shēng má	升麻		five fēn	1.85 g
mài mén dōng	麥門冬		five fēn	1.85 g
dāng guī shēn	當歸身		five fēn	1.85 g
shēng dì huáng	生地黃		five fēn	1.85 g
shén qū	神曲	stir-fried	five fēn	1.85 g
zhū líng	豬苓		five fēn	1.85 g
jiǔ bǎi	酒柏		five fēn	1.85 g
chái hú	柴胡		three fēn	1.11 g
huáng lián	黃連		three fēn	1.11 g
gān cǎo	甘草	mix-fried	three fēn	1.11 g

上薑水煎服。濕痰壅盛，參、耆、歸、地之類，可暫減之。

Boil the above in water with ginger and take it. Herbs like *rén shēn*, *huáng qí*, *dāng guī*, and *dì huáng* can be decreased temporarily for damp-phlegm congestion.

F-20 Shēng Mài Sǎn 生脈散
Pulse-Engendering Powder

治金瘡、杖瘡等症，發熱體倦，氣短；或汗多作渴；或潰後
睡臥不寧，陽氣下陷，發熱煩躁。若六七月間，濕熱大行，

火土合病，令人脾胃虛弱，身重氣短；或金為火制，絕寒水
化源，肢體痿軟，腳欹眼黑，並宜服。

Treats wounds inflicted by metal, wounds from caning, and similar conditions
with fever, weary body, and shortness of breath; or sweating copiously with
thirst; or sleep is not peaceful after [the wound] ulcerates and yáng qì sinks
downward, with fever, vexation, and agitation. If damp-heat strongly prevails
around the sixth or seventh month [July or August in the Western calendar],
the combined diseases of fire and earth makes people's spleen and stomach
deficient and weak with generalized heaviness and shortness of breath; or metal
is restrained by fire, severing the source of transformation for cold water, with
wěi-wilting and limpness of the body, crooked legs [slanting to one side], and
darkened vision. Taking this formula is appropriate for all of the above.

人參（ 五錢 ）五味子（ 一錢 ）麥門冬（ 一錢 ）

rén shēn	人參	five qián	18.65 g
wǔ wèi zǐ	五味子	one qián	3.73 g
mài mén dōng	麥門冬	one qián	3.73 g

用水煎服。

Boil in water and take it.

F-21 Èr Miào Wán 二妙丸
Two Marvels Pill

治下焦濕熱腫痛，或流注游走，遍身疼痛。

Treats damp-heat of the lower jiāo with swelling and pain; or streaming sores in
various places with pain of the entire body.

蒼朮黃柏（ 各等分 ）

| cāng zhú | 蒼朮 | equal portions of each |
| huáng bǎi | 黃柏 | |

117

用為末，每服二三錢，酒調服，作丸亦可 。

Use as a powder. Each dose is two or three *qián* (11.19 grams) mixed with liquor and taken; it can also be made into pills.

F-22 Sì Jīn Wán 四斤丸
Four Jīn Pill

治肝腎精血不足，筋無所養，攣縮不能步履，或邪淫於內，筋骨痿軟 。

Treats insufficient liver and kidney *jīng*-essence and blood so the sinews have nothing to nourish them, with contracture and inability to walk; or evil excesses on the interior with *wěi*-wilting and limpness of the sinews and bones.

肉蓯蓉（ 酒浸 ）牛膝（ 酒洗 ）天麻乾木瓜鹿茸（ 炙 ）熟地黃（ 生者自製 ）菟絲子（ 酒浸煮杵 ）五味子（ 各等分 ）

ròu cōng róng	肉蓯蓉	soaked in liquor	equal portions of each
niú xī	牛膝	washed in liquor	
tiān má	天麻		
gān mù guā	乾木瓜		
lù róng	鹿茸	mix-fried	
shú dì huáng	熟地黃	prepare it from the fresh yourself	
tú sī zǐ	菟絲子	wine soaked, boiled, and pestled	
wǔ wèi zǐ	五味子		

上為末，用地黃膏丸，桐子大 。每服五七十丸，空心溫酒送下 。

Powder the above. Make pills the size of *wú tóng zǐ* (about 0.6-0.9 centimeters in diameter) using *dì huáng* paste. Each dose is fifty or seventy pills, swallowed with warm liquor on an empty stomach.

118

F-23 Bǔ Zhōng Yì Qì Tāng 補中益氣湯
Center-Supplementing Qì-Boosting Decoction

治跌撲等症，損傷元氣，或過服克伐，惡寒發熱，肢體倦
怠，血氣虛弱，不能生肌收斂；或兼飲食勞倦，頭痛身熱，
煩躁作渴，脈洪大弦虛，或微細軟弱，自汗倦怠，飲食少
思。

Treats injuries from tumbles, beatings and similar conditions with injury to
original qì; or excessive doses of herbs that subdue and cut down with aversion to cold, fever, fatigued body, deficient weak blood and qì, and inability to
engender muscle or promote contraction; or simultaneous dietary [impro-
prieties] and taxation weariness with headache, generalized heat, vexation,
agitation, and thirst. The pulse is surging, large, bowstring, and deficient; or
faint, fine, soft, and weak with spontaneous sweating, fatigue, and little thought
of food and drink.

黃耆（炙）人參白朮甘草（炙，各一錢五分）當歸（一錢）
陳皮（五分）柴胡升麻（各三分）

huáng qí	黃耆	mix-fried	1.5 qián	1.85 g
rén shēn	人參		1.5 qián	1.85 g
bái zhú	白朮		1.5 qián	1.85 g
gān cǎo	甘草	mix-fried	1.5 qián	1.85 g
dāng guī	當歸		one qián	3.73 g
chén pí	陳皮		five fēn	1.85 g
chái hú	柴胡		three fēn	1.11 g
shēng má	升麻		three fēn	1.11 g

用薑棗水煎服。

Boil in water with ginger and *zǎo*-dates and take it.

F-24 Sì Shēng Sǎn 四生散
Four Fresh Agents Powder[67]

治腎臟風毒，遍身瘙癢，或膿水淋漓，耳鳴目癢，或鼻赤齒
浮，口舌生瘡。婦人血風瘡更效 。

Treats wind toxins of the kidney organ and itching of the entire body; or dripping pus-water with tinnitus and itching eyes; or red nose, loose teeth, and sores on the mouth and tongue. It is also effective for blood-wind sores in women.

白附子獨活黃耆蒺藜（ 各等分 ）

bái fù zǐ	白附子	equal portions of each
dú huó	獨活	
huáng qí	黃耆	
jí lí	蒺藜	

上為末，各等分，每服二錢，用腰子一枚，劈開入藥，濕紙
包裹，煨熟細嚼，鹽湯下，酒服亦可 。

Powder the above using equal portions of each. Each dose is two *qián* (7.46 grams). Split open a kidney[68] and put the herbs inside. Wrap it in moist paper, and roast until cooked. Chew it carefully and swallow it with hot salted water; it can also be taken with liquor.

F-25 Zhú Yè Huáng Qí Tāng 竹葉黃耆湯
Zhú Yè and Huáng Qí Decoction

治氣血虛，胃火盛，而作渴者 。

Treats qì and blood deficiency with abundance of stomach fire and thirst.

---

67. While these ingredients are dried so they can be powdered, they are not otherwise processed, hence the name.
68. *Nǔ Kē Cuò Yào* (Outline of Female Medicine) specifies pork kidney.

淡竹葉（ 二錢 ）黃耆生地黃當歸麥門冬川芎甘草黃芩（ 炒 ）
芍藥人參石膏（ 煅，各一錢 ）

dàn zhú yè	淡竹葉		two qián	7.46 g
huáng qí	黃耆		one qián	3.73 g
shēng dì huáng	生地黃		one qián	3.73 g
dāng guī	當歸		one qián	3.73 g
mài mén dōng	麥門冬		one qián	3.73 g
chuān xiōng	川芎		one qián	3.73 g
gān cǎo	甘草		one qián	3.73 g
huáng qín	黃芩	stir-fry	one qián	3.73 g
sháo yào	芍藥		one qián	3.73 g
rén shēn	人參		one qián	3.73 g
shí gāo	石膏	calcined	one qián	3.73 g

用水煎服 。

Boil in water and take it.

F-26 Zhú Yè Shí Gāo Tāng 竹葉石膏湯
Zhú Yè and Shí Gāo Decoction

治胃火盛，而作渴者 。

Treats abundance of stomach fire with thirst.

淡竹葉石膏（ 煅 ）桔梗木通薄荷甘草（ 各一錢 ）

dàn zhú yè	淡竹葉		one qián	3.73 g
shí gāo	石膏	calcined	one qián	3.73 g
jié gěng	桔梗		one qián	3.73 g
mù tōng	木通		one qián	3.73 g
bò hé	薄荷		one qián	3.73 g
gān cǎo	甘草		one qián	3.73 g

用薑水煎服 。

Boil in water with ginger and take it.

F-27 Rén Shēn Píng Fèi Yǐn 人參平肺飲
Rén Shēn Lung-Calming Drink[69]

治心火克肺，咳嗽喘嘔，痰涎壅盛，咽喉不利等症 。

Treats heart fire controlling the lungs with cough, wheezing, retching, phlegm-drool congestion, inhibited throat, and similar conditions.

人參陳皮甘草（ 各一錢 ）地骨皮茯苓知母（ 各八分 ）五味子
青皮天門冬桑白皮（ 各五分 ）

rén shēn	人參	one qián	3.73 g
chén pí	陳皮	one qián	3.73 g
gān cǎo	甘草	one qián	3.73 g
dì gǔ pí	地骨皮	eight fēn	2.96 g
fú líng	茯苓	eight fēn	2.96 g
zhī mǔ	知母	eight fēn	2.96 g
wǔ wèi zǐ	五味子	five fēn	1.85 g
qīng pí	青皮	five fēn	1.85 g
tiān mén dōng	天門冬	five fēn	1.85 g
sāng bái pí	桑白皮	five fēn	1.85 g

上水煎服 。

Boil the above in water and take it.

---

69. This formula is also called *Rén Shēn Píng Fèi Sǎn* 人參平肺散 (Rén Shēn Lung-Calming Powder). In fact, the author himself calls it that in the text.

F-28 Zī Shèn Wán 滋腎丸
Kidney-Enriching Pill

治腎經陰虛，發熱作渴，足熱，腿膝無力等症。凡不渴而小
便閉者，最宜用之。

Treats yīn deficiency of the kidney channel with fever, thirst, hot feet, feeble legs and knees, and similar conditions. Whenever the patient is not thirsty and urination is blocked, it is especially suitable to use this.

肉桂（ 三錢 ）知母（ 酒炒 ）黃柏（ 酒炒，各二兩 ）

ròu guì	肉桂		three qián	11.19 g
zhī mǔ	知母	stir-fried with liquor	two liǎng	74.6 g
huáng bǎi	黃柏	stir-fried with liquor	two liǎng	74.6 g

上為末，水丸，桐子大。每服七八十丸，空心白滾湯下。

Powder the above. Make water pills the size of *wú tóng zǐ* (about 0.6-0.9 centimeters in diameter). Each dose is seventy or eighty pills taken on an empty stomach and swallowed with plain boiled water.

F-29 Liù Wèi Dì Huáng Wán 六味地黃丸
Six Ingredient Dì Huáng Pill

加肉桂、五味各一兩，名加減八味丸。

Adding one *liǎng* (37.3 grams) each of *ròu guì* and *wǔ wèi zǐ* is named F-29a *Jiā Jiǎn Bā Wèi Wán* (Eight Ingredient Variant Pill).

治傷損之症，因腎肺二經虛弱，發熱作渴，頭暈眼花，咽燥
唇裂，齒不堅固，腰腿痿軟，小便頻赤，自汗盜汗，便血
諸血，失喑，水泛為痰之聖藥。血虛發熱之神劑。若損重傷
骨，不能言如喑者，用此水煎服之，亦效。

Treats injury conditions due to deficiency and weakness of both the kidney and lung channels, with fever, thirst, dizzy head, blurry vision, dry throat, cracked lips, loose teeth, *wěi*-wilting and limpness of the lower back and legs, frequent red urination, spontaneous sweating, night sweating, bloody stool, all bleeding disorders, loss of voice, water overflowing and becoming phlegm; it is sagacious medicine. It is a divine prescription for blood deficiency fevers. If the injury is severe with damaged bones and inability to speak as if mute, boil this in water and take it; it is also effective.

熟地黃（ 八兩，杵膏自製 ）山茱萸肉乾山藥（ 各四兩 ）牡丹皮白茯苓澤瀉（ 各三兩 ）

shú dì huáng	熟地黃	pestle into a paste, prepare it yourself	eight liǎng	298.4 g
shān zhū yú ròu	山茱萸肉		four liǎng	149.2 g
gān shān yào	乾山藥		four liǎng	149.2 g
mǔ dān pí	牡丹皮		three liǎng	111.9 g
bái fú líng	白茯苓		three liǎng	111.9 g
zé xiè	澤瀉		three liǎng	111.9 g

上為末，和地黃丸桐子大。每服七八十丸，空心食前滾湯下。

Powder the above. Blend with the *dì huáng* paste to make pills the size of *wú tóng zǐ* (about 0.6-0.9 centimeters in diameter). Each dose is seventy or eighty pills taken before meals on an empty stomach. Swallow them with boiled water.

F-30 Qīng Xīn Lián Zǐ Yǐn 清心蓮子飲
Heart-Clearing Lián Zǐ Drink

治發熱口渴白濁，夜安靜而晝發熱等症 。

Treats fever, thirst, and white turbidity when the patient is peaceful at night but feverish in the daytime, and similar conditions.

黃芩（ 一錢 ）麥門冬地骨皮車前子（ 炒 ）甘草（ 各一錢五分 ）石蓮肉茯苓黃耆（ 炒 ）柴胡人參（ 各一錢 ）

huáng qín	黃芩		one qián	3.73 g
mài mén dōng	麥門冬		1.5 qián	5.6 g
dì gǔ pí	地骨皮		1.5 qián	5.6 g
chē qián zǐ	車前子	stir-fry	1.5 qián	5.6 g
gān cǎo	甘草		1.5 qián	5.6 g
shí lián ròu	石蓮肉		one qián	3.73 g
fú líng	茯苓		one qián	3.73 g
huáng qí	黃耆	stir-fry	one qián	3.73 g
chái hú	柴胡		one qián	3.73 g
rén shēn	人參		one qián	3.73 g

上水煎服 。

Boil the above in water and take it.

F-31 Qī Wèi Bái Zhú Sǎn 七味白朮散
Seven Ingredient Bái Zhú Powder

治脾胃虛弱，津液短少，口乾作渴，或中風虛熱，口舌生
瘡，不喜飲冷 。最宜服之 。

Treats deficiency and weakness of the spleen and stomach with scant *jīnyè*-
fluids, dry mouth, and thirst; or wind strike with deficiency heat, sores on the
mouth and tongue, and dislike of cold drinks. It is especially appropriate to take
this.

人參白朮木香白茯苓甘草（ 炙 ）藿香（ 各五分 ）乾葛（ 一
錢 ）

rén shēn	人參		five fēn	1.85 g
bái zhú	白朮		five fēn	1.85 g
mù xiāng	木香		five fēn	1.85 g
bái fú líng	白茯苓		five fēn	1.85 g
gān cǎo	甘草	mix-fried	five fēn	1.85 g
huò xiāng	藿香		five fēn	1.85 g
gān gé	乾葛		one qián	3.73 g

用水煎服 。

Boil in water and take it.

F-32 Hēi Wán Zǐ 黑丸子
Black Pill

一名和血定痛丸 。

Another name is F-32 *Hé Xuè Dìng Tòng Wán* (Blood-Harmonizing Pain-Settling Pill).

治跌撲墜墮，筋骨疼痛，或瘀血壅腫，或風寒肢體作痛 。若流注膝風初結，服之自消 。若潰而膿清發熱，與補氣血藥，兼服自斂 。

Treats injuries from tumbles, beatings, and falls with pain of the sinews and bones; or blood stasis with congestion and swelling; or wind-cold in the body causing pain. During the initial onset of streaming sores or knee wind, taking this will automatically disperse it. If there are ulcerations with clear pus and fever, take it along with herbs to supplement qì and blood and they will close up without further intervention.

百草霜白芍藥（ 各一兩 ）赤小豆（ 一兩六錢 ）川烏（ 炮，三錢 ）白蘞（ 一兩六錢 ）白芨當歸（ 各八錢 ）南星（ 泡，三錢 ）牛膝（ 焙，六錢 ）骨碎補（ 焙，六錢 ）

bǎi cǎo shuāng	百草霜		one liǎng	37.3 g
bái sháo yào	白芍藥		one liǎng	37.3 g
chì xiǎo dòu	赤小豆		1.6 liǎng	59.68 g
chuān wū	川烏	blast-fried	three qián	11.19 g
bái liǎn	白蘞		1.6 liǎng	59.68 g
bái jī	白芨		eight qián	29.84 g
dāng guī	當歸		eight qián	29.84 g
nán xīng	南星	soaked	three qián	11.19 g
niú xī	牛膝	stone-baked	six qián	22.38 g
gǔ suì bǔ	骨碎補	stone-baked	six qián	22.38 g

上各另為末，酒糊丸，桐子大，每服三十丸，鹽湯溫酒送
下 。孕婦勿服 。

Powder each of the above separately; make it into pills the size of *wú tóng zǐ*
(about 0.6-0.9 centimeters in diameter) with paste made from wheat and
liquor. Each dose is thirty pills swallowed with hot salted water or warm liquor.
Pregnant women should not take it.

F-33 Bái Wán Zǐ 白丸子
White Pill[70]

治一切風痰壅盛，手足頑麻，或牙關緊急，口眼歪斜，半身
不遂等症 。

Treats all types of wind-phlegm congestion with stubborn numbness of the
hands and feet; or clenched jaw, deviation of the mouth and eyes, half-body
paralysis, and similar conditions.

半夏（七兩，生用 ）南星（ 二兩，生用 ）川烏（ 生用，去皮
臍，五錢 ）

bàn xià	半夏	use the fresh	seven liǎng	261.1 g
nán xīng	南星	use the fresh	two liǎng	74.6 g
chuān wū	川烏	use the fresh, remove the skin and 'umbilicus'	five qián	18.65 g

上為末，用生薑汁調糊丸，桐子大 。每服一二十丸，薑湯送
下 。

Powder the above. Make pills the size of *wú tóng zǐ* (about 0.6-0.9 centimeters
in diameter) by mixing with paste made from wheat and ginger juice. Each
dose is ten or twenty pills, swallowed with a decoction of ginger.

---

70. This formula probably could not be used today in the West due to toxicity. It is
identical to F-73 *Bái Wán Zǐ*.

F-34 Liù Jūn Zǐ Tāng 六君子湯
Six Gentlemen Decoction

治金瘡、杖瘡等症，因元氣虛弱，腫痛不消，或不潰斂，或
服克伐傷脾，或不思飲食，宜服之以壯營氣。

Treats wounds inflicted by metal, wounds from caning, and similar conditions
when swelling and pain does not disperse due to deficiency and weakness of
original qì; or wounds that do not ulcerate and close up; or there is injury to the
spleen from taking herbs that subdue and cut down; or no thought of food and
drink. It is appropriate to take this to invigorate *yíng* qì.

此方即四君子湯，加陳皮、白朮。

This formula is F-1 *Sì Jūn Zǐ Tāng* adding *chén pí* and *bái zhú*.

更加香附、藿香、砂仁，香砂六君子。

Further adding *xiāng fù, huò xiāng*, and *shā rén* is F-34a *Xiāng Shā Liù Jūn Zǐ Tāng*
(Fragrant Shā Rén Six Gentlemen Decoction).

F-35 Huí Yáng Yù Lóng Gāo 回陽玉龍膏
Yáng-Returning Jade Dragon Paste

治跌撲所傷，為敷涼藥，或人元氣虛寒，腫不消散，或不潰
斂，及癰腫堅硬，肉色不變，久而不潰，潰而不斂，或筋攣
骨痛，一切冷症並效。

Treats injury from tumbles and beatings when cooling herbs were applied; or
the patient's original qì is deficient and cold so the swelling does not disperse;
or it doesn't ulcerate and close up until it becomes a swollen hard abscess. The
color of the flesh does not change and it lasts for a long time without ulcerating
or it ulcerates but does not close up; or there is hypertonicity of the sinews with
bone pain. It is equally effective for all types of cold conditions.

草烏（ 二錢 ）南星（ 一兩，煅 ）軍薑（ 炒，一兩 ）白芷（ 一兩 ）赤芍藥（ 一兩，炒 ）肉桂（ 五錢 ）

cǎo wū	草烏		two qián	7.46 g
nán xīng	南星	calcined	one liǎng	37.3 g
jūn jiāng	軍薑	stir-fry	one liǎng	37.3 g
bái zhǐ	白芷		one liǎng	37.3 g
chì sháo yào	赤芍藥	stir-fry	one liǎng	37.3 g
ròu guì	肉桂		five qián	18.65 g

用為末，蔥湯調塗，熱酒亦可 。

Use as a powder mixed with a decoction of scallions. Smear it on. Hot liquor can also be used [instead of the scallion decoction].

F-36 Fù Yuán Huó Xuè Tāng 復原活血湯
Source-Restoring Blood-Quickening Decoction

治跌撲等症，瘀血停凝，脅腹作痛，甚者大便不通 。

Treats tumbles, beatings, and similar conditions when there is blood stasis collecting and congealing with pain in the rib-sides and abdomen. When serious, there is constipation.

柴胡當歸紅花（ 各二錢 ）穿山甲（ 炮，五分 ）大黃（ 酒炒，一錢 ）桃仁（ 二十枚 ）甘草（ 五分 ）瓜蔞根（ 一錢 ）

chái hú	柴胡		two qián	7.46 g
dāng guī	當歸		two qián	7.46 g
hóng huā	紅花		two qián	7.46 g
chuān shān jiǎ*	穿山甲	blast-fried	five fēn	1.85 g
dà huáng	大黃	stir-fried with liquor	one qián	3.73 g
táo rén	桃仁			twenty pieces
gān cǎo	甘草		five fēn	1.85 g
guā lóu gēn	瓜蔞根		one qián	3.73 g

* *Chuān shān jiǎ* is from an endangered animal so it cannot be used today.

129

用酒水各半煎服 。

Boil in half each of liquor and water and take it.

F-37 Fù Yuán Tōng Qì Sǎn 復原通氣散
Source-Restoring Qì-Freeing Decoction

治打撲傷損作痛，及乳癰便毒初起，或氣滯作痛 。

Treats injury from a beating with pain, as well as breast abscess and inguinal toxins[71] when they initially arise; or qì stagnation with pain.

木香茴香（ 炒 ）青皮（ 去白 ）穿山甲（ 酥炙 ）陳皮白芷甘草 漏蘆貝母（ 各等分 ）

mù xiāng	木香		equal portions of each
huí xiāng	茴香	stir-fry	
qīng pí	青皮	remove the white	
chuān shān jiǎ*	穿山甲	mix-fried with shortening	
chén pí	陳皮		
bái zhǐ	白芷		
gān cǎo	甘草		
lòu lú	漏蘆		
bèi mǔ	貝母		

* *Chuān shān jiǎ* is from an endangered animal so it cannot be used today.

上為末，每服一二錢，溫酒調下 。

Powder the above. Each dose is one or two *qián* (7.46 grams) mixed with warm liquor and swallowed.

---

71. *Biàn dú* 便毒 (inguinal toxins): This may be inguinal buboes in the Western medical paradigm.

愚按：前方治打撲閃挫或惱怒，氣滯血凝作痛之良劑。

I humbly note: The above formulas [F-35 through F- 37] are good prescriptions to treat injuries from beatings, wrenching, and contusions; perhaps the patient is furious, and qì stagnation and congealed blood cause pain.

經云：形傷作痛，氣傷作腫。又云：先腫而後痛者，形傷氣也；先痛而後腫者，氣傷形也。

The Classic says: Injury to the physical body makes pain; injury to qì makes swelling. It also says: If swelling manifests first and pain comes later, it means the physical body has injured qì; if pain manifests first and swelling comes later, it means qì has injured the physical body.[72]

若人元氣素弱，或因叫號，血氣損傷，或過服克伐之劑，或外敷寒涼之藥，血氣凝結者。當審前大法，用溫補氣血為善。

Blood congeals and qì binds if a person's original qì is usually weak; perhaps blood and qì are injured due to yelling; or excessively taking prescriptions to subdue and cut down; or external application of cold and cool medicine. One should examine the above fundamental methods and consider it good to use herbs that warm and supplement qì and blood.

F-38 Shén Xiào Tài Yǐ Gāo 神效太乙膏
Wondrous Effect Tài Yǐ Ointment

治癧疽、發背、杖瘡，及一切瘡疽潰爛。

---

72. This is paraphrased from *Sù Wèn • Yīn Yáng Yìng Xiàng Dà Lùn*, Chapter 5, which says: "氣傷痛，形傷腫。故先痛而後腫者，氣傷形也；先腫而後痛者，形傷氣也。 Injury to qì is pain, injury to the physical body is swelling. Thus, if pain manifests first and swelling comes later, it means qì has injured the physical body; if swelling manifests first and pain comes later, it means the physical body has injured qì." Note that Xuē's text partially disagrees with *Sù Wèn*. Is it a typo? Did he remember it wrong? Or did he change it on purpose? We do not know.

Treats abscesses, eruptions on the back, and wounds from caning, as well as all types of festering wounds or abscesses.

玄參白芷當歸肉桂赤芍藥大黃生地黃（ 各一兩 ）

xuán shēn	玄參	one liǎng	37.3 g
bái zhǐ	白芷	one liǎng	37.3 g
dāng guī	當歸	one liǎng	37.3 g
ròu guì	肉桂	one liǎng	37.3 g
chì sháo yào	赤芍藥	one liǎng	37.3 g
dà huáng	大黃	one liǎng	37.3 g
shēng dì huáng	生地黃	one liǎng	37.3 g

用麻油二斤，入銅鍋內煎至藥黑，濾去渣，徐入淨黃丹十二兩，再煎，滴水中捻軟硬得中，即成膏矣 。

Put two *jīn* (1.193 kilograms) of sesame oil [along with the above herbs] into a copper wok and boil until the herbs turn black; filter to remove the dregs. Slowly add in twenty *liǎng* (746 grams) of clean *huáng dān*[73] and boil again. Drip some into water and then rub it between your fingers to see if the correct degree of hardness or softness is obtained, meaning it has become an ointment.[74]

F-39 Rǔ Xiāng Dìng Tòng Sǎn 乳香定痛散
Rǔ Xiāng Pain-Settling Powder

治杖瘡 、金瘡，及一切瘡瘍，潰爛疼痛 。

Treats wounds from caning and wounds inflicted by metal, as well as all types of sores that are festering and painful.

---

73. *Huáng dān* 黃丹 is minium or red lead. It is not considered appropriate today due to toxicity, even for external use. The rest of the herbs in this formula are acceptable so the ointment could be thickened with beeswax instead.

74. The ointment is dripped into water to cool it rapidly. When it is rubbed between the fingers, the maker can decide when it is the proper viscosity.

乳香沒藥（ 各五錢 ）滑石（ 一兩 ）寒水石（ 一兩，煅 ）冰片
（ 一錢 ）

rǔ xiāng	乳香		five qián	18.65 g
mò yào	沒藥		five qián	18.65 g
huá shí	滑石		one liǎng	37.3 g
hán shuǐ shí	寒水石	calcined	one liǎng	37.3 g
bīng piàn	冰片		one qián	3.73 g

上為末，搽患處，痛即止，甚效 。

Powder the above. Rub it into the affected site. The pain will stop; it is extremely effective.

F-40 Zhū Tí Tāng 豬蹄湯
Pig Hoof Decoction

治一切癰疽 、杖瘡潰爛，消腫毒，去惡肉 。

Treats all types of abscesses and festering wounds from caning; it disperses
swellings and toxins and removes malign flesh.

白芷當歸羌活赤芍藥露蜂房（ 蜂兒多者佳 ）生甘草（ 各五
錢 ）

bái zhǐ	白芷		five qián	18.65 g
dāng guī	當歸		five qián	18.65 g
qiāng huó	羌活		five qián	18.65 g
chì sháo yào	赤芍藥		five qián	18.65 g
lù fēng fáng	露蜂房	good quality has a lot of wasp larvae	five qián	18.65 g
shēng gān cǎo	生甘草		five qián	18.65 g

用豬蹄一只，水五碗，煮熟取清湯，入前藥，煎數沸去渣，
溫洗，隨用膏藥貼之 。

133

Boil one pig's hoof in five bowlfuls of water until cooked; reserve the clear broth. Add in the above herbs, boil for several boilings,[75] and remove the dregs. Use it as a warm wash. Follow up by sticking on an herbal plaster.

F-41 Shén Xiào Dāng Guī Gāo 神效當歸膏
Wondrously Effective Dāng Guī Ointment

治杖撲湯火瘡毒，不問已潰未潰，肉雖傷而未壞者，用之自癒。肉已死而用之自潰，新肉易生。搽至肉色漸白，其毒始盡，生肌最速。

Treats toxins from wounds after canings, beatings, scalds, or burns; don't bother to ask if the wound has ulcerated or not. Even if the flesh is injured but has not yet disintegrated, it will automatically recover when this is used. If the flesh is already dead, it will automatically ulcerate when used and new flesh will easily grow. Rub it in until the color of the flesh gradually whitens[76] and the toxins begin to exhaust themselves; the growth of muscle will be very quick.

如棍杖者，外皮不破，肉內糜爛，其外皮因內燉乾縮，堅硬不潰，爬連好肉作痛。故俗云丁痂皮，致膿瘀無從而泄，內愈脹痛，腐潰益深，往往不待其潰，就行割去，而瘡口開張，難以潰斂。怯弱之人，多成破傷風症，每致不救。

If beaten with a rod or cane, the skin may not break open on the outside but inside the flesh is reduced to a pulp. The skin outside is dry and withered due to internal scorching; it becomes hard and does not ulcerate. [The damage] creeps into the good flesh, causing pain. Thus it is commonly called *scabbed skin*. The result is that pus and stasis have no way to drain out so there is more

---

75. In the ancient past, sometimes formulas were said to be boiled for a number of boilings. This means to bring the decoction to a boil, add a ladle of room temperature water, and bring it to a boil again. This would be repeated the specified number of times. Here, an exact number was not given, but perhaps this was done three or five times.
76. The injured flesh would be red, purple, or dark, depending on the condition. Whitens indicates that the flesh will return to its original color.

distention and pain internally, with increasingly deep putrid ulceration. One often cannot wait for it to ulcerate, and it approaches the need for surgical removal; the opening of the wound expands and it becomes difficult for the ulceration to close. In a weak person, it often develops into the condition of tetanus; whenever this occurs, the result is that he cannot be rescued.

若杖瘡內有瘀血者，即用有鋒芒磁片，於患處砭去，塗以此藥，則丁痂自結，死肉自潰，膿穢自出，所潰亦淺，生肌之際，亦不結痂，又免皴揭之痛，殊有神效 。

If there is internal blood stasis due to wounds from caning, *biān*-lance the affected site with the sharp edge of a porcelain shard and remove the stasis. When this medicine is smeared on, the scab will automatically form, the dead flesh will automatically ulcerate, and the pus and foulness will automatically exude. The area that ulcerates will also be shallow; it will grow muscle on the border and it will not form a scab. The pain of chapping due to exposure will also be avoided. This formula has especially divine effects.

蓋當歸、地黃、麻油、二蠟，主生肌止痛，補血續筋，與新肉相宜 。此方余以刊行，治者亦多用之 。

It seems that *dāng guī*, *dì huáng*, sesame oil, and the two waxes [white and yellow wax] are indicated for engendering muscle, stopping pain, supplementing blood, and joining sinews. It is suitable for producing new flesh. I publish this formula, as many others also use it.

當歸（ 一兩 ）麻油（ 六兩 ）黃蠟（ 一兩 ）生地黃（ 一兩 ）

dāng guī	當歸	one liǎng	37.3 g
má yóu	麻油	six liǎng	223.8 g
yellow wax (huáng là)	黃蠟	one liǎng	37.3 g
shēng dì huáng	生地黃	one liǎng	37.3 g

上先將當歸、地黃入油煎黑去粗，入蠟溶化，候冷攪勻，即成膏矣 。白蠟尤效 。

From the above, first put the *dāng guī* and *dì huáng* into the oil and boil them until they are blackened. Remove the dregs. Add the wax and let it dissolve. Wait for it to cool, stirring evenly until it becomes an ointment. White wax (*bái là*) is especially effective.

F-42 Tuō Lǐ Sǎn 托裏散
Draw Out the Interior Powder[77]

治金瘡、杖瘡，及一切瘡毒。因氣血虛不能成膿，或膿成不能潰斂，膿水清稀，久而不瘥。

Treats wounds inflicted by metal or wounds from caning, as well as toxins from all types of sores or wounds. This is due to qì and blood deficiency with inability to form pus; or pus forms but the wound is unable to ulcerate and close up, with clear thin pus-water that lasts for a long time without recuperating.

人參（一錢，氣虛多用之）黃耆（鹽水拌炒，一兩）白朮（炒）陳皮（各七分）當歸身（酒拌，一錢）芍藥（酒炒）熟地黃（生者，自製）白茯苓（各一錢）

rén shēn	人參	use more for qì deficiency	one qián	3.73 g
huáng qí	黃耆	mix with salty water and stir-fry	one liǎng	37.3 g
bái zhú	白朮	stir-fry	seven fēn	2.59 g
chén pí	陳皮		seven fēn	2.59 g
dāng guī shēn	當歸身	mix with liquor	one qián	3.73 g
sháo yào	芍藥	stir-fried with liquor	one qián	3.73 g
shú dì huáng	熟地黃	prepare it from the fresh yourself	one qián	3.73 g
bái fú líng	白茯苓		one qián	3.73 g

用水煎服。

Boil in water and take it.

---

77. *Tuō lǐ* 托裏 (drawing out the interior): Also translated as *internal expression*. This is the treatment method of pushing toxins (including their manifestation as pus) outward from the inside of the body by supplementing right qì.

F-43 Jiā Wèi Xiōng Guī Tāng 加味芎歸湯
Supplemented Chuān Xiōng and Dāng Guī Decoction

治跌撲墜墮，皮膚不破，瘀血入胃作嘔。

Treats injuries from tumbles, beatings, and falls when the skin is not broken and blood stasis enters the stomach, with vomiting.

芎窮當歸百合（水浸半日）白芍藥荊芥穗（各二錢）

xiōng qióng	芎窮		two qián	7.46 g
dāng guī	當歸		two qián	7.46 g
bǎi hé	百合	soak in water for half a day*	two qián	7.46 g
bái sháo yào	白芍藥		two qián	7.46 g
jīng jiè suì	荊芥穗		two qián	7.46 g

* This word for *day* means a twenty-four hour period (not daytime), so one would soak it for about twelve hours.

用酒水煎服。

Boil it in liquor and water and take it.

F-44 Dāng Guī Dǎo Zhì Sǎn 當歸導滯散
Dāng Guī Powder to Lead out Stagnation

治跌撲，瘀血在內，胸腹脹滿，或大便不通，或喘咳吐血。

Treats tumbles and beatings when there is internal blood stasis, with distension and fullness of the chest and abdomen; or constipation; or panting, coughing, and spitting blood.

大黃當歸（各等分）

dà huáng	大黃	equal portions of each
dāng guī	當歸	

用為末，每服三錢，溫酒下。氣虛須加桂。

Use as a powder. Each dose is three *qián* (11.19 grams) swallowed with warm liquor. *Guì*-cinnamon must be added for qì deficiency.

F-45 Huā Ruǐ Shí Sǎn 花蕊石散
Huā Ruǐ Shí Powder[78]

治打撲傷損，腹中瘀血，脹痛欲死，服之血化為水，其功不能盡述。

Treats injury from a beating when there is blood stasis in the abdomen, with distention and pain, and the patient is about to die. Taking it makes the blood [stasis] transform into water; its achievements cannot all be recounted.

硫黃（明色者，四兩）花蕊石（一兩）

| liú huáng | 硫黃 | bright colored | four liǎng | 149.2 g |
| huā ruǐ shí | 花蕊石 | | one liǎng | 37.3 g |

上為末和勻。先用紙筋和鹽泥固濟瓦罐一個，候乾入藥，再用泥封口，安在磚上，虛書八卦五行，用炭三十斤煅之，罐冷取出。每服一錢，童便調下。

Powder the above and blend evenly. First use strips of paper and a slurry of salt and mud to make an earthen jar; wait for it to dry and put the herbs in it. Then use mud to seal the opening, Set it on bricks. Write the characters for the eight *guà* and five elements in the air.[79] Use thirty *jīn* (about 18 kilograms) of charcoal to calcine [the jar of minerals]. When the jar is cool, take out the contents.[80] Each dose is one *qián* (3.73 grams) mixed with child's urine and swallowed.

---

78. This is probably unacceptable for use today.
79. This empowers the herbs with some magic.
80. *Nǚ Kē Cuò Yào* (Summary of Female Medicine) says to then powder the minerals.

愚按：前方若被傷熾盛，元氣虧損，內有瘀血，不勝疏導
者，用前藥一服，其血內化，又不動臟腑，甚妙、甚妙！

I humbly note: For the above formula, if the injury causes vigorous blazing, enfeebled original qì, and blood stasis inside [under the skin], but he cannot physically bear treatment to course and lead it out, use one dose of the above herbs; the blood will transform internally and in addition, it will not stir up the *zàngfǔ*-organs. It is extremely effective! It is extremely effective!

F-46 Jīng Yàn Fāng 經驗方
Empirical Formula

治跌撲瘀血作痛，或筋骨疼痛。

Treats tumbles and beatings with blood stasis and pain; or pain of the sinews and bones.

黃柏（ 一兩 ）半夏（ 五錢 ）

| huáng bǎi | 黃柏 | one liǎng | 37.3 g |
| bàn xià | 半夏 | five qián | 18.65 g |

上為末，用薑汁調塗患處，以紙貼之，如乾，薑汁潤之，周
日易之。

Powder the above. Mix with ginger juice and smear it on the affected site. Use paper to stick it on. If it dries, moisten it with ginger juice. Change it once a day.

F-47 Xiāo Dú Dìng Tòng Sǎn 消毒定痛散
Toxin-Dispersing Pain-Settling Powder

治跌撲腫痛。

Treats tumbles and beatings with swelling and pain.

無名異（ 炒 ）木耳（ 炒 ）大黃（ 炒，各五分 ）

wú míng yì	無名異	pyrolusite	stir-fry	five fēn	1.85 g
mù ěr	木耳		stir-fry	five fēn	1.85 g
dà huáng	大黃		stir-fry	five fēn	1.85 g

上為末，蜜水調塗 。如內有瘀血，砭去敷之 。若腐處，更用
當歸膏敷之尤妙 。

Powder the above. Mix with honey and water and smear it on. If there is blood
stasis inside [under the skin], *biān*-lance to remove it and apply this. If the site
has putrefied, further apply F-41 *Dāng Guī Gāo* to it; this is especially wonderful.

F-48 Yào Qū Fāng 藥蛆方
Herbal Maggot Formula

治杖瘡潰爛生蛆 。

Treats festering wounds with maggots from caning.

用皂礬煅過為末乾摻，其內蛆即死 。如未應，佐以柴胡梔子
散，以清肝火 。

Powder *zào fán* (melanterite) that has been calcined and sprinkle the dry powder [on the wounds]. The maggots inside will die. If there is no response, assist
by using UF-9 *Chái Hú Zhī Zǐ Sǎn* to clear liver fire.

F-49 Xǐ Yào 洗藥
Herbal Wash

凡傷重者，用此淋洗，然後敷藥。

Whenever there is serious injury, drip-wash the wound with this; afterwards apply herbs externally.

荊芥土當歸生蔥（ 切斷，一方用生薑 ）

jīng jiè	荊芥		
tǔ dāng guī	土當歸		
shēng cōng	生蔥	fresh scallions	cut off the ends; one formula book uses shēng jiāng

上煎湯溫洗，或止用蔥一味，煎洗亦可。

Decoct the above to make a warm wash. Or only use the cōng (scallions) alone; you can also boil them and wash with it.

F-50 Hēi Lóng Sǎn 黑龍散
Black Dragon Powder

治跌撲傷損，筋骨碎斷。先用前湯淋洗，以紙攤貼。若骨折，更以薄木片夾貼，以小繩束三日，再如前法。勿去夾板，恐搖動患處，至骨堅牢，方宜去。

Treats injuries from tumbles and beatings with shattered or severed sinews and bones. First use the previous decoction [F-49 Xǐ Yào] to drip-wash; stick this powder on paper then apply it [on the affected site]. If a bone is broken, further use thin wooden strips to squeeze [the limb], sticking the strips on and binding them with thin rope for three days. Again use the above method. Do not remove the splint or else you risk jostling the affected site. Only when the bones are firm and fast is it appropriate to remove the splints.

141

若被刀箭蟲傷成瘡，並用薑汁和水調貼，口以風流散填塗 。

If an injury from knives, arrows, or *chóng*-worms[81] develops into a wound, mix this powder with ginger juice blended with water and stick it on; at the same time smear UF-10 *Fēng Liú Sǎn* at the opening [of the wound] to fill it in.

土當歸（ 二兩 ）丁香皮（ 六兩 ）百草霜（ 散血，入六兩 ）穿
山甲（ 六兩，炒黃或煉存性 ）枇杷葉（ 去毛，入半兩，一云
山枇杷根 ）

tǔ dāng guī	土當歸		two liǎng	74.6 g
dīng xiāng pí	丁香皮		six liǎng	223.8 g
bǎi cǎo shuāng	百草霜	dissipates blood [stasis]	add in six liǎng	223.8 g
chuān shān jiǎ˙	穿山甲	stir-fry until yellow or process preserving its nature[†]	six liǎng	223.8 g
pí pá yè	枇杷葉	remove the hairs, one source says to use shān pí pá gēn	half a liǎng	18.65 g

* *Chuān shān jiǎ* is from an endangered animal so it cannot be used today.

†This means it is processed using heat but not to the point where it is totally charred.

上焙為細末，薑汁水調 。或研地黃汁調，亦好 。

Stone-bake the above and make into a fine powder; mix with ginger juice and water. Or it is also good to grind [fresh] *dì huáng* for its juice and mix that with the powder.

F-51 Hóng Bǎo Dān 洪寶丹
Vast Treasure Elixir

一名濟陰丹

Another name is F-51 *Jì Yīn Dān* (Yīn-Saving Elixir)

治傷損焮痛，並接斷 。

Treats injuries with scorching pain and rejoins severed [sinews or bones].

81. The word *chóng* 蟲 has a much broader range of meaning then worms in English. It can include snakes, bugs, reptiles, and the like (creepy-crawlies), as well as some invisible disease-causing entities. *Chóng*-worms may be visible or invisible.

天花粉（　三兩　）薑黃白芷赤芍藥（　各一兩　）

tiān huā fěn	天花粉	three liǎng	111.9 g
jiāng huáng	薑黃	one liǎng	37.3 g
bái zhǐ	白芷	one liǎng	37.3 g
chì sháo yào	赤芍藥	one liǎng	37.3 g

上為末，茶湯調搽患處。

Powder the above. Mix with a decoction of tea and rub it onto the affected site.

F-52 [Unnamed Formula A]

治金傷出血不止。用牛膽、石灰，摻之即止。以臘月牛膽入風化石灰，懸當風，候乾用。

Treats wounds inflicted by metal with bleeding that does not stop. Sprinkle on *niú dǎn*[82] and *shí huī* and it will stop. Add *niú dǎn* that was gathered in the twelfth lunar month (*là yuè*) into *fēng huà shí huī* (air-slaked lime). Suspend it in the wind, wait until dry, and use.

F-53 Yòu Fāng 又方
Another [Unnamed] Formula B

金瘡出血不止，以五倍子生為末，乾貼。

For wounds inflicted by metal with bleeding that won't stop: Powder fresh *wǔ bèi zǐ* and stick it on dry.

如不止，屬血熱，宜用犀角地黃湯之類。

If the bleeding doesn't stop, it belongs to blood heat; it is appropriate to use formulas like F-5 *Xī Jiǎo Dì Huáng Tāng*.[83]

---

82. This is bile from an ox or cow, although the term can also mean the gall bladder of an ox or cow.
83. This cannot be used today as *xī jiǎo* is from an endangered species.

143

大凡金瘡出血不止，若素怯弱者，當補氣。若素有熱，當補血。若因怒氣，當平肝。若煩熱作渴昏憒，當補脾氣。若筋攣搐搦，當養肝血。不應，用地黃丸，以滋腎水。

Generally speaking, for wounds inflicted by metal with bleeding that won't stop:

▸ If the patient is usually physically weak, one should supplement qì.

▸ If the patient is usually hot, one should supplement blood.

▸ If it is due to anger, one should calm the liver.

▸ If there is vexation heat, thirst, and he is in a daze, one should supplement spleen qì.

▸ If there is hypertonicity of the sinews and convulsions, one should nourish liver blood.

▸ If he does not respond, use F-29 *Dì Huáng Wán* to enrich kidney water.

F-54 Yòu Fāng 又方
Another [Unnamed] Formula C

皮破筋斷者，以百膠香塗之，或以金沸草汁頻塗，自然相續。

For broken skin and severed sinews, smear *bǎi jiāo xiāng* on it; or frequently smear *jīn fèi cǎo* juice on it. They will naturally reconnect.

F-55 Mò Yào Jiàng Shèng Dān 沒藥降聖丹
Mò Yào Descending Sage Elixir

治傷損筋骨疼痛，或不能屈伸，肩背拘急，身體倦怠，四肢無力。

Treats injury to sinews and bones with pain; or inability to bend and extend with hypertonicity of the shoulders and upper back, fatigued body, and feeble limbs.

沒藥（別研）當歸（酒洗，炒）白芍藥骨碎補（撏去毛）川烏（去毛臍，泡）川芎（各一兩半）自然銅（火煅醋淬十二次，研為末，水飛過，焙，一兩）

mò yào	沒藥	grind separately	1.5 liǎng	55.95 g
dāng guī	當歸	wash with liquor, stir-fry	1.5 liǎng	55.95 g
bái sháo yào	白芍藥		1.5 liǎng	55.95 g
gǔ suì bǔ	骨碎補	pluck out the hairs	1.5 liǎng	55.95 g
chuān wū	川烏	remove the hairs and 'umbilicus,' soak	1.5 liǎng	55.95 g
chuān xiōng	川芎		1.5 liǎng	55.95 g
zì rán tóng	自然銅	calcine in fire and quench in vinegar twelve times, grind into powder, stone-bake after water grinding	one liǎng	37.3 g

上為細末，每一兩作四丸，以生薑自然汁與煉蜜為丸。每服一丸，搥碎，用水酒各半鐘，入蘇木少許，煎至八分，去蘇木，空心服。

Make the above into a fine powder. Each one *liǎng* (37.3 grams) of the powder makes four pills. Make the pills with the natural juice of fresh ginger and processed honey. Each dose is one pill. [At the time of use,] pound the pill into pieces. Use a half cup each of water and liquor, add in a little *sū mù*, and boil until it is eighty percent of the original. Remove the *sū mù* and take it on an empty stomach.

愚按：脾主肉，肝主筋。若因肝脾二經氣血虛弱，或血虛有熱而不愈者，當求其本而治之。

I humbly note: The spleen governs flesh; the liver governs sinews. If the patient doesn't recover and the condition is due to qì and blood deficiency of both the liver and spleen channels or blood deficiency with heat; one should treat it by seeking the root.

F-56 Wàn Jīn Gāo 萬金膏
Unlimited Gold Plaster

治癰疽及墜撲傷損，或筋骨疼痛 。

Treats abscesses as well as injuries from falls and beatings, or pain of the sinews and bones.

龍骨鱉甲苦參烏賊魚骨黃柏黃芩黃連白芨白蘞豬牙皂角厚朴草烏川芎當歸木鱉子仁白芷（ 各一兩 ）沒藥（ 另研 ）乳香（ 另研，各半兩 ）槐枝柳枝（ 各四寸長，二十一條 ）黃丹（ 一斤半，炒過淨 ）清油（ 四斤 ）

lóng gǔ	龍骨		one liǎng	37.3 g
biē jiǎ	鱉甲		one liǎng	37.3 g
kǔ shēn	苦參		one liǎng	37.3 g
wū zéi yú gǔ	烏賊魚骨		one liǎng	37.3 g
huáng bǎi	黃柏		one liǎng	37.3 g
huáng qín	黃芩		one liǎng	37.3 g
huáng lián	黃連		one liǎng	37.3 g
bái jī	白芨		one liǎng	37.3 g
bái liǎn	白蘞		one liǎng	37.3 g
zhū yá zào jiǎo	豬牙皂角		one liǎng	37.3 g
hòu pǔ	厚朴		one liǎng	37.3 g
cǎo wū	草烏		one liǎng	37.3 g
chuān xiōng	川芎		one liǎng	37.3 g
dāng guī	當歸		one liǎng	37.3 g
mù biē zi rén	木鱉子仁		one liǎng	37.3 g
bái zhǐ	白芷		one liǎng	37.3 g
mò yào	沒藥	grind separately	a half liǎng	18.65 g
rǔ xiāng	乳香	grind separately	a half liǎng	18.65 g
huái zhī	槐枝		21 four cùn lengths	
liǔ zhī	柳枝		21 four cùn lengths	
huáng dān*	黃丹	clean after stir-frying	1.5 jīn	895.2 g
qīng yóu	清油		four jīn	2387.2 g

* *Huáng dān* is minium or red lead. It is not considered appropriate today due to toxicity, even for external use. The ointment could be thickened with beeswax instead.

上除乳、沒、黃丹外，諸藥入油內，煎至黑色去之，稱淨
油，每斤入丹半斤，不住手攪令黑色，滴水中不粘手，下
乳、沒再攪，如硬，入油些少，以不粘手為度。

Put all the above herbs except *rǔ xiāng, mò yào*, and *huáng dān* into the oil. Boil until they are blackened and remove them. Weigh the clean oil [after the dregs are filtered out]; for each *jīn* (596.8 grams) of oil, add a half *jīn* (298.4 grams) of *huáng dān*. Do not stop stirring or else it will turn black. Drip some of the ointment into water and when it does not stick to the hand,[84] add the *rǔ xiāng* and *mò yào* and stir again. If it is too hard, add a little more oil. Not being sticky is the goal.

F-57 Jiē Gǔ Sǎn 接骨散
Bone-Joining Powder

治骨折碎，或骨出骱，先整端正，卻服此藥。如飛禽六畜所
傷，亦能治。

Treats broken or shattered bones; or the bone has come out of its socket [dislocation]. First adjust the ends so they are straight [set the bone or reduce the dislocation], then take this medicine. It is also able to treat birds or livestock that are injured.

硼砂（ 一錢五分 ）水粉當歸（ 各一錢 ）

péng shā	硼砂	1.5 qián	5.6 g
shuǐ fěn	水粉	one qián	3.73 g
dāng guī	當歸	one qián	3.73 g

上為末，每服二錢，煎蘇木湯調服，後但飲蘇木湯，立效。

Powder the above. Each dose is two *qián* (7.46 grams). Boil it in a decoction of *sū mù*, mix, and take it. Afterwards only drink *sū mù* decoction; it is immediately effective.

---

84. A little is dripped into water to cool it. It is tested by feeling it for the proper texture.

F-58 Běn Shì Jiē Gǔ Fāng 《本事》接骨方
Bone-Joining Formula from Běn Shì[85]

治打折傷損。

Treats injury from beatings or breaks.

接骨木（半兩，即蒴藋也）乳香（半兩）赤芍藥當歸川芎自然銅（各一兩）

jiē gǔ mù	接骨木	this means shuò liǎo	half liǎng	18.65 g
rǔ xiāng	乳香		half liǎng	18.65 g
chì sháo yào	赤芍藥		one liǎng	37.3 g
dāng guī	當歸		one liǎng	37.3 g
chuān xiōng	川芎		one liǎng	37.3 g
zì rán tóng	自然銅		one liǎng	37.3 g

上為末，用黃蠟四兩溶入前末攪勻，眾手丸龍眼大。如打傷筋骨及閃痛不堪忍者，用一丸，熱酒浸開熱呷，痛便止。若大段傷損，先整骨，用川烏、草烏等分為末，生薑汁調貼之。挾定服藥，無不效者。

Powder the above. Add four *liǎng* (149.2 grams) of melted yellow wax into the above powder and mix evenly. Have many people make pills the size of *lóng yǎn*.[86] When a beating has injured the sinews and bones, as well as for unendurable pain from wrenching, soak one pill in hot liquor to open it, and sip it while hot; the pain will then stop. If a large section [of the bone] is injured, first right [set] the bone, powder equal portions of *chuān wū* and *cǎo wū*, mix with ginger juice, and stick it on. Clasp it firmly [with splints] and take these herbs; they never fail to be effective.

---

85. *Běn Shì* 《本事》 refers to *Pǔ Jì Běn Shì Fāng* 許叔微《普濟本事方》宋 by·Xǔ Shūwēi (*Sòng*).
86. Since the pills are made with melted wax, unless they are quickly formed, the wax will become unworkable. Many people can make the batch of pills more quickly.

愚按：前三方俱效者備錄之，以便修用 。

I humbly note: The above three formulas [F-56, F-57, and F-58] are all effective. I fully recorded them so that they could be studied for use.

F-59 Mò Yào Wán 沒藥丸
Mò Yào Pill

治打撲筋骨疼痛，或血逆血暈，或瘀血內停，肚腹作痛，或
胸膈脹悶 。

Treats pain of the sinews and bones from a beating; or blood counterflow with blood dizziness; or blood stasis collecting on the interior with bellyache; or distention and oppression of the chest and diaphragm.

沒藥乳香川芎川椒芍藥當歸桃仁血竭（ 各一兩 ）自然銅（ 四
錢，火煅七次 ）

mò yào	沒藥		one liǎng	37.3 g
rǔ xiāng	乳香		one liǎng	37.3 g
chuān xiōng	川芎		one liǎng	37.3 g
chuān jiāo	川椒		one liǎng	37.3 g
sháo yào	芍藥		one liǎng	37.3 g
dāng guī	當歸		one liǎng	37.3 g
táo rén	桃仁		one liǎng	37.3 g
xuè jié	血竭		one liǎng	37.3 g
zì rán tóng	自然銅	calcine in fire seven times	four qián	14.92 g

上為末，用黃蠟四兩，溶化入前末，速攪勻，丸彈子大 。每
服一丸，酒化服 。

Powder the above. Add four *liǎng* (149.2 grams) of melted yellow wax into the above powder and quickly mix evenly. Make pills the size of slingshot pellets. Each dose is one pill. Dissolve it in liquor and take it.

愚按：接骨散 、沒藥丸，元氣無虧者，宜用 。若腎氣素怯，
或高年腎氣虛弱者，必用地黃丸 、補中益氣湯，以固其本為
善 。

I humbly note: F-57 *Jiē Gǔ Sǎn* and F-59 *Mò Yào Wán* are suitable to use when
original qì is not lacking. If kidney qì is usually weak, or there is kidney qì
deficiency in an older person, it is good to use F-29 *Dì Huáng Wán* or F-23 *Bǔ
Zhōng Yì Qì Tāng* to secure the root.

F-60 Qiāng Huó Fáng Fēng Tāng 羌活防風湯
Qiāng Huó and Fáng Fēng Decoction

治破傷風，邪初在表者，急服此藥以解之 。稍遲則邪入於
裏，與藥不相合矣 。

Treats tetanus when evils are initially located in the exterior; quickly take this
medicine to resolve it. When you are a little late, evils enter the interior, which is
incompatible with these herbs.

羌活防風甘草川芎藁本當歸芍藥（ 各四兩 ）地榆細辛（ 各二
兩 ）

qiāng huó	羌活	four liǎng	149.2 g
fáng fēng	防風	four liǎng	149.2 g
gān cǎo	甘草	four liǎng	149.2 g
chuān xiōng	川芎	four liǎng	149.2 g
gǎo běn	藁本	four liǎng	149.2 g
dāng guī	當歸	four liǎng	149.2 g
sháo yào	芍藥	four liǎng	149.2 g
dì yú	地榆	two liǎng	74.6 g
xì xīn	細辛	two liǎng	74.6 g

上每服五錢，水煎 。

Each dose of the above is five *qián* (18.65 grams), boiled in water.

F-61 Fáng Fēng Tāng 防風湯
Fáng Fēng Decoction

治破傷風，表症未傳入裏，急宜服之 。

Treats tetanus in exterior conditions that have not yet transmitted to the interior; it is appropriate to quickly take this.

防風羌活獨活川芎（ 各等分 ）

fáng fēng	防風	equal portions of each
qiāng huó	羌活	
dú huó	獨活	
chuān xiōng	川芎	

上每服五錢，水煎，調蜈蚣散服，大效 。

Each dose of the above is five *qián* (18.65 grams), boiled in water. When mixed with F-62 *Wú Gōng Sǎn* and taken, it is very effective.

F-62 Wú Gōng Sǎn 蜈蚣散
Wú Gōng Powder

蜈蚣（ 一對 ）鰾（ 三錢 ）

wú gōng	蜈蚣	a pair	
biào	鰾	three qián	11.19 g

上為細末，用防風湯調下 。

Make the above into a fine powder, mix with F-61 *Fáng Fēng Tāng*, and swallow it.

F-63 Qiāng Huó Tāng 羌活湯
Qiāng Huó Decoction

治破傷風，在半表半裏，急用此湯。稍緩邪入於裏，不宜用。

Treats tetanus located half in the exterior and half in the interior; quickly use this decoction. If you are a little late, evils enter into the interior and then this not appropriate to use.

羌活菊花麻黃川芎石膏防風前胡黃芩細辛甘草白茯苓枳殼蔓荊子（各一兩）薄荷白芷（各五錢）

qiāng huó	羌活	one liǎng	37.3 g
jú huā	菊花	one liǎng	37.3 g
má huáng	麻黃	one liǎng	37.3 g
chuān xiōng	川芎	one liǎng	37.3 g
shí gāo	石膏	one liǎng	37.3 g
fáng fēng	防風	one liǎng	37.3 g
qián hú	前胡	one liǎng	37.3 g
huáng qín	黃芩	one liǎng	37.3 g
xì xīn	細辛	one liǎng	37.3 g
gān cǎo	甘草	one liǎng	37.3 g
bái fú líng	白茯苓	one liǎng	37.3 g
zhǐ qiào	枳殼	one liǎng	37.3 g
màn jīng zǐ	蔓荊子	one liǎng	37.3 g
bò hé	薄荷	five qián	18.65 g
bái zhǐ	白芷	five qián	18.65 g

上每服五錢，水煎。

Each dose of the above is five *qián* (18.65 grams), boiled in water.

F-64 Dì Yú Fáng Fēng Sǎn 地榆防風散
Dì Yú and Fáng Fēng Powder

治風在半表半裏，頭微汗，身無汗，不可發汗，兼治表裏。

Treats wind located half in the exterior and half in the interior with slight sweating on the head but no sweating on the body. One cannot promote sweating. This simultaneously treats the exterior and interior.

地榆防風地丁草馬齒莧（ 各等分 ）

dì yú	地榆	equal portions of each
fáng fēng	防風	
dì dīng cǎo	地丁草	
mǎ chǐ xiàn	馬齒莧	

上為細末，每服三錢，米湯調服。

Make the above into a fine powder. Each dose is three *qián* (11.19 grams); mix with water in which rice was cooked and take it.

F-65 Dà Xiōng Huáng Tāng 大芎黃湯
Major Chuān Xiōng and Yellows Decoction

治風在裏，宜疏導，急服此湯。

Treats wind located in the interior. It is appropriate to course and lead it out; quickly take this decoction.

川芎羌活黃芩大黃（ 各一兩 ）

chuān xiōng	川芎	one liǎng	37.3 g
qiāng huó	羌活	one liǎng	37.3 g
huáng qín	黃芩	one liǎng	37.3 g
dà huáng	大黃	one liǎng	37.3 g

153

上五七錢，水煎溫服，臟腑通利為度 。

Boil five or seven *qián* of the above in water and take it warm. The goal is free-flowing disinhibited *zàngfǔ*-organs.

F-66 Bái Zhú Fáng Fēng Tāng 白朮防風湯
Bái Zhú and Fáng Fēng Decoction[87]

治服表藥過多自汗者 。

Treats spontaneous sweating after taking excessive amounts of herbs for the exterior.

白朮黃耆（ 各一兩 ）防風（ 二兩 ）

báizhú	白朮	one liǎng	37.3 g
huáng qí	黃耆	one liǎng	37.3 g
fáng fēng	防風	two liǎng	74.6 g

上每服五七錢，水煎服 。臟腑和而自汗者可服 。若臟腑秘，小便赤者，宜用大芎黃湯下之 。

Each dose of the above is five to seven *qián*. Boil in water and take it. It can be taken when the *zàngfǔ*-organs are harmonious but there is spontaneous sweating. If the *zàngfǔ*-organs are hoarding [constipated] and there is red urine, it is appropriate to use F-65 *Dà Xiōng Huáng Tāng* to descend it [promote a bowel movement].

---

87. These three ingredients are more commonly known as *Yù Píng Fēng Sǎn* 玉屏風散 (Jade Wind Screen Powder) although the dosage of each herb is different.

F-67 Bái Zhú Tāng 白朮湯
Bái Zhú Decoction

治破傷風汗不止，筋攣搐搦。

Treats tetanus with incessant sweating, hypertonicity of the sinews, and convulsions.

白朮葛根升麻黃芩芍藥（ 各二兩 ）甘草（ 二錢五分 ）

bái zhú	白朮	two liǎng	74.6 g
gé gēn	葛根	two liǎng	74.6 g
shēng má	升麻	two liǎng	74.6 g
huáng qín	黃芩	two liǎng	74.6 g
sháo yào	芍藥	two liǎng	74.6 g
gān cǎo	甘草	2.5 qián	9.33 g

上每服五錢，水煎，無時服。

Each dose of the above is five *qián* (18.65 grams) boiled in water. Take at any time.

F-68 Qiān Fǔ Zhū Shā Wán 謙甫朱砂丸
Qiānfǔ's Zhū Shā Pill[88]

治破傷風，目瞪口噤不語，手足搐搦，項筋強直，不能轉側，目不識人。

Treats tetanus, with staring eyes, clenched jaw with inability to speak, convulsions of the hands and feet, rigidity of the sinews at the nape, inability to turn to the sides, and inability of the eyes to recognize people.

---

88. This formula is not appropriate for use today. Luó Qiānfǔ 羅謙甫 was a *Yuán* dynasty doctor. Xuē Jǐ specified in the title of the formula that this is Luó's version of *Zhū Shā Wán*.

朱砂（ 研 ）半夏（ 洗 ）川烏（ 各一兩 ）雄黄（ 五錢 ）鳳凰臺
（ 三錢 ）麝香（ 一字 ）

zhū shā	朱砂	grind	one liǎng	37.3 g
bàn xià	半夏	wash	one liǎng	37.3 g
chuān wū	川烏		one liǎng	37.3 g
xióng huáng	雄黃		five qián	18.65 g
fèng huáng tái	鳳凰臺		three qián	11.19 g
shè xiāng	麝香		one zì*	

*Zì 字 is an ancient measurement. There are four characters (zì 字) written on one side of the old coins that have a square hole in the center. One zì is as much herbal powder as it takes to cover one of the characters.

上為末，棗肉丸，桐子大 。每服一丸或二丸，冷水下，以吐
為度 。如不吐，加一丸 。或吐不住，煎蔥白湯止之 。汗出為
效 。

Powder the above. Make pills the size of *wú tóng zǐ* (about 0.6-0.9 centimeters in diameter) with *zǎo*-date flesh. Each dose is one or two pills swallowed with cold water. Take vomiting as the goal. If the patient does not vomit, add another pill. Or if vomiting doesn't cease, boil a decoction of *cōng bái* to stop it. It is effective when the patient sweats.

F-69 Zuǒ Lóng Wán 左龍丸
Left Dragon Pill

治直視在裏者 。

Treats forward-staring eyes from [tetanus] in the interior.

左盤龍（ 野鴿糞 ）白僵蠶鰾（ 炒，各五錢 ）雄黃（ 一錢 ）

zuǒ pán lóng	左盤龍	[this is another name for] yě gē fèn	five qián	18.65 g
bái jiāng cán	白僵蠶		five qián	18.65 g
biào	鰾	stir-fry	five qián	18.65 g
xióng huáng	雄黃		one qián	3.73 g

上為末，燒飯丸，桐子大 。每服十五丸，溫酒下 。

Powder the above. Make pills the size of *wú tóng zǐ* (about 0.6-0.9 centimeters in diameter) with cooked rice. Each dose is fifteen pills swallowed with warm liquor.

如裏症不已，當用前藥末一半，加巴豆霜半錢，燒飯丸，桐子大 。每服加入一丸，如此漸加，以利為度 。利後服和解藥 。

If the interior condition does not cease, a half *qián* (1.87 grams) of *bā dòu shuāng* should be added to one half of the above herbal powder. Make pills the size of *wú tóng zǐ* (about 0.6-0.9 centimeters in diameter) with cooked rice. Add in one pill [with *bā dòu shuāng*] to each dose [of the original formula], gradually increasing like this. Take disinhibition as the goal.[89] After disinhibition, take harmonizing herbs.

F-70 Jiāng Biào Wán 江鰾丸
Jiāng Biào Pill

治破傷風，傳入裏症，驚而發搐，臟腑秘澀 。

Treats tetanus that has been transmitted into the interior with fright and jerking, when the *zàng fǔ*-organs are hoarding and astringed [no urination or bowel movement].

江鰾（ 銼炒，半兩 ）野鴿糞（ 炒，半兩 ）雄黃（ 一錢 ）白僵蠶（ 半兩 ）蜈蚣（ 一對 ）天麻（ 一兩 ）

jiāng biào	江鰾	grate and stir-fry it	half liǎng	18.65 g
yě gē fèn	野鴿糞	stir-fry	half liǎng	18.65 g
xióng huáng	雄黃		one qián	3.73 g
bái jiāng cán	白僵蠶		half liǎng	18.65 g

89. The function of *bā dòu shuāng* is to drastically descend. It promotes forceful diarrhea and expulsion of urine, here called 'disinhibiton.' Once this occurs, its use should be stopped. It is the same for the next formula, F-70 *Jiāng Biào Wán*.

| wú gōng | 蜈蚣 | | a pair | |
| tiān má | 天麻 | | one liǎng | 37.3 g |

上為末，作三分；二分，燒飯丸，桐子大，朱砂為衣；一分，入巴豆霜一錢，亦用燒飯丸。每服朱砂者二十丸，入巴豆者一丸，漸加至利為度，後止服前丸。

Powder the above. Divide it into three portions. Make two portions into pills the size of *wú tóng zǐ* (about 0.6-0.9 centimeters in diameter) with cooked rice and coat them with *zhū shā*.[90] Add one *qián* (3.73 grams) of *bā dòu shuāng* to the other portion and make pills again with cooked rice. Each dose is twenty pills with *zhū shā*, adding in one pill with *bā dòu*. Gradually increase [the *bā dòu* pills] until disinhibition occurs as the goal; after this, only take the previous pill [the one without *bā dòu*].

F-71 Yǎng Xuè Dāng Guī Dì Huáng Tāng 養血當歸地黃湯
Blood-Nourishing Dāng Guī and Dì Huáng Decoction

當歸地黃芍藥川芎藁本防風白芷（各一兩）細辛（五錢）

dāng guī	當歸	one liǎng	37.3 g
dì huáng	地黃	one liǎng	37.3 g
sháo yào	芍藥	one liǎng	37.3 g
chuān xiōng	川芎	one liǎng	37.3 g
gǎo běn	藁本	one liǎng	37.3 g
fáng fēng	防風	one liǎng	37.3 g
bái zhǐ	白芷	one liǎng	37.3 g
xì xīn	細辛	five qián	18.65 g

上依前煎服。

The above are boiled and taken the same way as the previous formulas.

---

90. *Zhū shā* cannot be used today due to its potential toxicity.

F-72 Guǎng Lì Fāng 廣利方
Guǎng Lì Formula[91]

治破傷風發熱 。

Treats tetanus with fever.

瓜蔞子（九錢）滑石（三錢半）南星蒼朮赤芍藥陳皮炒柏黃
連黃芩白芷甘草（各五分）

guā lóu zǐ	瓜蔞子	nine qián	33.57 g
huá shí	滑石	3.5 qián	13.06 g
nán xīng	南星	five fēn	1.85 g
cāng zhú	蒼朮	five fēn	1.85 g
chì sháo yào	赤芍藥	five fēn	1.85 g
chén pí	陳皮	five fēn	1.85 g
chǎo bǎi	炒柏	five fēn	1.85 g
huáng lián	黃連	five fēn	1.85 g
huáng qín	黃芩	five fēn	1.85 g
bái zhǐ	白芷	five fēn	1.85 g
gān cǎo	甘草	five fēn	1.85 g

用薑水煎服 。

Boil in water with ginger and take it.

上二方，用竹瀝 、瓜蔞實輩，治破傷風熱痰脈洪者 。前方用
南星 、半夏 、草烏 、川烏輩，則治破傷風寒痰脈無力者 。

▶ Use herbs like *zhú lì* and *guā lóu shí* with the above two formulas to treat tetanus with hot phlegm and a surging pulse.
▶ Use herbs like *nán xīng, bàn xià, cǎo wū,* and *chuān wū* with the previous
formulas to treat tetanus with cold phlegm and a forcelss pulse.

---

91. *Zhēn Yuán Guǎng Lì Fāng* 《貞元廣利方》 is the name of a *Táng* dynasty formula book. Here, the name is shortened to *Guǎng Lì Fāng.*

F-73 Bái Wán Zǐ 白丸子
White Pill[92]

治一切風痰壅盛，手足頑麻，或牙關緊急，口眼歪斜，半身
不遂等症。

Treats all types of wind-phlegm congestion with stubborn numbness of the
hands and feet, or clenched jaw, deviation of the mouth and eyes, half-body
paralysis, and similar conditions.

半夏（ 七兩，生用 ）南星（ 二兩，生用 ）川烏（ 去皮臍，生
用，五錢 ）

bàn xià	半夏	use the fresh	seven liǎng	261.1 g
nán xīng	南星	use the fresh	two liǎng	74.6 g
chuān wū	川烏	remove the skin and umbilicus, use the fresh	five qián	18.65 g

上為末，用生薑汁調糊丸，桐子大。每服一二十丸，薑湯
下。

Powder the above. Make pills the size of *wú tóng zǐ* (about 0.6-0.9 centimeters
in diameter) by mixing with wheat paste made using ginger juice. Each dose is
ten or twenty pills, swallowed with a decoction of ginger.

F-74 Běn Shì Yù Zhēn Sǎn 《本事》玉真散
True Jade Powder from Běn Shì

治破傷風，及打撲損傷，項強口噤欲死。

Treats tetanus, as well as injury from a beating with neck rigidity and clenched
jaw when the patient is about to die.

---

92. This probably could not be used today in the West due to toxicity. This formula is
identical to F-33 *Bái Wán Zǐ*.

南星有防風制其毒，不麻人。

The toxins of nán xīng are controlled by fáng fēng, so it won't make the patient numb.

天南星（ 湯泡七次 ）防風（ 等分 ）

tiān nán xīng	天南星	soak in hot water seven times	equal portions
fáng fēng	防風		

上為末，先以熱童子小便洗淨瘡口，拭乾摻之，良久渾身作癢，瘡口出赤水是效 。又以溫酒調下一錢 。如牙關緊急，腰背反張，用藥二錢，童子小便調服 。至死心頭微溫者，急灌之，亦可救，累效累驗 。

Powder the above. First use hot child's urine to clean the opening of the wound, wipe it dry and sprinkle the powder on. There will be itching from head to foot for a good long time. It is effective when red water comes out from the opening of the wound. Then mix one *qián* (3.73 grams) of the powder with warm liquor and swallow it. If the jaw is clenched and there is arched-back rigidity, take two *qián* (7.46 grams) mixed with child's urine. If the patient has died but the heart and head are slightly warm, quickly pour it in and you still can save them. It is repeatedly effective and repeatedly proven.

F-75 [Unnamed Formula D]

治打撲傷損，腫痛傷風者 。

Treats injury from a beating with swelling, pain, or wind damage.

天南星半夏地龍（ 各等分 ）

tiān nán xīng	天南星	equal portions of each
bàn xià	半夏	
dì lóng	地龍	

上為末，用生薑、薄荷汁，調搽患處。

Powder the above. Mix with the juices of *shēng jiāng* and *bò hé* and rub it into the affected site.

Appendix

Unlisted Formulas Recommended by Xuē Jǐ

These formulas were mentioned in the text as being useful, but were not included with the formulas given in Volume Two. Perhaps in the pre-computer age, it was harder to keep track of all the formulas suggested in the text. While they generally have earlier sources than the ones I give below, most of the recipes here were taken from other books written or edited by Xuē Jǐ. In this way, we can be assured that the version of the formula presented here would be the one that Xuē Jǐ had in mind. Note that the indications listed may be influenced by the topic of the source book. For example, if a formula below was taken from one of Xuē Jǐ's books on gynecology, it may list more symptoms related to women's health.

UF-1 Jiā Wèi Xiāo Yáo Sǎn 加味逍遙散
Supplemented Free Wanderer Powder

治血虛有熱，遍身瘙癢；或口燥咽乾，發熱盜汗，食少嗜臥，小便澀滯等症 。

Treats blood deficiency with heat and itching of the entire body; or dry throat and mouth, fever, night sweating, decreased food intake, somnolence, rough stagnant bowel movement, and similar conditions.

甘草（ 炙 ）當歸（ 炒 ）芍藥（ 酒炒 ）茯苓白朮（ 炒 ）柴胡（ 各一錢 ）牡丹皮山梔（ 炒 。各五分 ）

gān cǎo	甘草	mix-fried	one qián	3.73 g
dāng guī	當歸	stir-fried	one qián	3.73 g
sháo yào	芍藥	stir-fried with liquor	one qián	3.73 g
fú líng	茯苓		one qián	3.73 g
bái zhú	白朮	stir-fried	one qián	3.73 g
chái hú	柴胡		one qián	3.73 g
mǔ dān pí	牡丹皮		five fēn	1.85 g
shān zhī zǐ	山梔	stir-fried	five fēn	1.85 g

上水煎服 。

Boil the above in water and take it.

Source: Volume 2 of *Nǚ Kē Cuò Yào* 《女科撮要》 by Xuē Jǐ 薛己 *Míng* (明).

UF-2 Fù Zǐ Sì Nì Tāng 附子四逆湯
Fù Zǐ Counterflow Cold Decoction

傷寒寒結膀胱，臍似冰，飲水下焦聲瀝瀝，主脈沉，客脈滑者 。

Treats cold damage with cold binding the urinary bladder, the umbilicus feels like ice, and there are trickling sounds in the lower jiāo after drinking water. The host pulse is sunken; the guest pulse is slippery.

炮附子半兩，炮薑半兩，白朮一兩，甘草三錢，桂七錢

pào fù zǐ	炮附子	a half liǎng	18.65 g
pào jiāng	炮薑	a half liǎng	18.65 g
bái zhú	白朮	one liǎng	37.3 g
gān cǎo	甘草	three qián	11.19 g
guì-cinnamon	桂	seven qián	287.2 g

上㕮咀 。每服一兩，水二盞，煎至一盞，去滓，食前溫服 。

Break the above into coarse pieces. Each dose is one *liǎng* (37.3 grams) in two small-cups of water boiled down to one small-cup. Remove the dregs. Take warm before meals.

Source: *Yún Qí Zǐ Mài Jué* 《雲岐子脈訣》 by Zhāng Bì 張璧 *Yuán* (元).[93]

---

93. There is uncertainty about which formula was meant by Xuē Jǐ. In the text, Xuē appears to attribute *Fù Zǐ Sì Nì Tāng* to *Wài Tái Mì Yào* 《外臺秘要》. Searching through it, *Sì Nì Tāng* was mentioned there a few times, but not *Fù Zǐ Sì Nì Tāng*. *Sì Nì Tāng* contains *fù zǐ*, *pào jiāng*, and *gān cǎo*. It was first described in *Shāng Hán Lùn*. This *Fù Zǐ Sì Nì Tāng* has a few additional ingredients.

UF-3 Èr Chén Tāng 二陳湯
Two Matured Ingredients Decoction

治脾虛，中脘停痰，嘔吐惡心，或頭目不清，飲食少思等症 。

Treats spleen deficiency with phlegm collecting at *zhōng wǎn* (the center of the stomach or the name of Rèn 12), vomiting, and nausea; or lack of clarity in the head and eyes, little thought of food and drink, and similar conditions.

陳皮半夏茯苓（ 各一錢 ）甘草（ 炙五分 ）

chén pí	陳皮		one qián	3.73 g
bàn xià	半夏		one qián	3.73 g
fú líng	茯苓		one qián	3.73 g
gān cǎo	甘草	mix-fried	five fēn	1.85 g

上薑水煎 。

Boil the above in water with ginger.

Source: Volume 4 of *Wài Kē Shū Yào* 《 外科樞要 》 by Xuē Jǐ 薛己 *Míng* (明).

UF-4 Jiā Wèi Sì Jūn Zǐ Tāng 加味四君子湯
Supplemented Four Gentlemen Decoction

即前方四君子湯加川芎 、當歸 。

This means the above formula, F-1 *Sì Jūn Zǐ Tāng* adding *chuān xiōng* and *dāng guī*.

Source: Volume 24 of *Xiào Zhù Fù Rén Liáng Fāng* 《 校注婦人良方 》 by Xuē Jǐ 薛己 *Míng* (明).

UF-5 Tiáo Zhōng Yì Qì Tāng 調中益氣湯
Center-Attuning Qì-Boosting Decoction

治體怠嗜臥，不思飲食；或痰嗽泄瀉等症 。

Treats body fatigue with somnolence and no thought of food or drink, or phlegm cough, diarrhea, and similar conditions.

黃耆（ 一錢 ）人參（ 去蘆頭 ）甘草蒼朮（ 各五分 ）柴胡橘皮
升麻木香（ 各二分 ）

huáng qí	黃耆		one qián	3.73 g
rén shēn	人參	remove the stem and head	five fēn	1.85 g
gān cǎo	甘草		five fēn	1.85 g
cāng zhú	蒼朮		five fēn	1.85 g
chái hú	柴胡		two fēn	0.74 g
jú pí	橘皮		two fēn	0.74 g
shēng má	升麻		two fēn	0.74 g
mù xiāng	木香		two fēn	0.74 g

上薑棗水煎，空心服 。

Boil the above in water with ginger and zǎo-dates and take it on an empty stomach.

Source: Volume 1 of *Nǚ Kē Cuò Yào* 《 女科撮要 》 by Xuē Jǐ 薛己 *Míng* (明)

UF-6 Qīng Shǔ Yì Qì Tāng 清暑益氣湯
Summerheat-Clearing Qì-Boosting Decoction

治元氣弱，暑熱乘之，精神困倦，胸滿氣促，肢節疼痛；或
小便黃數，大便溏頻 。又暑熱瀉痢瘧疾之良劑 。

Treats the heat of summer taking advantage of weak original qì with fatigued *jīng-shén*, chest fullness, hasty breathing, and pain in the joints of the limbs; or frequent yellow urination and frequent sloppy stool. It is also a good prescription for diarrhea and *nüè*-malarial disease during the heat of summer.

升麻黃耆（炒，去汗，各一錢）蒼朮（一錢五分）人參白朮
陳皮神曲（炒，各五分）甘草（炙）乾葛（各三分）五味子
（九粒，杵炒）

shēng má	升麻		one qián	3.73 g
huáng qí	黃耆	stir-fry to remove the 'sweat'	one qián	3.73 g
cāng zhú	蒼朮		1.5 qián	5.6 g
rén shēn	人參		five fēn	1.85 g
bái zhú	白朮		five fēn	1.85 g
chén pí	陳皮		five fēn	1.85 g
shén qū	神曲	stir-fry	five fēn	1.85 g
gān cǎo	甘草	mix-fried	three fēn	1.11 g
gàn gé	乾葛		three fēn	1.11 g
wǔ wèi zǐ	五味子	pestle, stir-fry		nine pieces

上水煎服 。

Boil the above in water and take it.

Source: Volume 2 of *Nǚ Kē Cuò Yào* 《 女科撮要 》 by Xuē Jǐ 薛己 *Míng* (明)

UF-7 Gé Gēn Tāng 葛根湯
Gé Gēn Decoction

治天時炎熱，欲發痘瘡，服此解肌發表 。

Treats heavenly seasonal blazing heat, about to erupt in pox sores. Taking this resolves the flesh and effuses the exterior.

赤芍藥石膏（火煅）乾葛甘草（炙，各五錢）黃芩（五錢）

chì sháo yào	赤芍藥		five qián	18.65 g
shí gāo	石膏	calcine with fire	five qián	18.65 g

gān gé	乾葛		five qián	18.65 g
gān cǎo	甘草	mix-fried	five qián	18.65 g
huáng qín	黄芩		five qián	18.65 g

上剉，葱白、薄荷湯煎，乳後服 。一方止用水煎 。無汗，加
麻黄；自汗，加桂皮 。

Cut up the above and decoct with *cōng bái* and *bò hé*. Take after milk. One
formula only uses water to boil it. If there is no sweating, add *má huáng*; if there
is spontaneous sweating, add *guì pí*.

Source: Volume 403 of *Pǔ Jì Fāng* 《 普濟方 》 by Zhū Sù 朱橚 1406, *Míng* (明).[94]

UF-8 Xiāo Yáo Sǎn 逍遙散
Free Wanderer Powder

治婦人血虛，五心煩熱，肢體疼痛，頭目昏重，心忪頰赤，
口燥咽乾，發熱盜汗，食少嗜臥，及血熱相搏，月水不調，
臍服脹痛，寒熱如虐，及至室女血弱，榮衛不調，痰嗽潮
熱，肌體羸瘦，漸成骨蒸 。

Treats blood deficiency in women with five heart vexation heat, painful body,
clouded heavy head and eyes, palpitations, red cheeks, dry mouth and throat,
fever, night sweating, decreased food intake, and somnolence; or blood and
heat mingled with each other, irregular menstruation, distending pain in the
umbilical region and abdomen, and *nüè*-malaria-like chills and fever; or weak
blood in unmarried girls, disharmony of *yíng* and *wèi*, phlegmy cough, tidal
fever, and emaciated body that gradually develops into steaming bones.

當歸（ 酒拌 ）芍藥茯苓白朮（ 炒 ）柴胡（ 各一錢 ）甘草（ 七
分 ）

---

94. I could not find a version of *Gé Gēn Tāng* in Xuē Jǐ's books. This formula origi-
nated in *Shāng Hán Lùn*, but one can find more than fifty variations in later books. So it
is quite possible that Xuē had a different variation in mind when he recommended this
formula, but we do not know which one.

dāng guī	當歸	mixed with liquor	one qián	3.73 g
sháo yào	芍藥		one qián	3.73 g
fú líng	茯苓		one qián	3.73 g
bái zhú	白朮	stir-fried	one qián	3.73 g
chái hú	柴胡		one qián	3.73 g
gān cǎo	甘草		seven fēn	2.59 g

作一劑，水二鐘，煎八分，食遠服 。

This makes one dose. Boil in two cups of water down to eighty percent. Take between meals.

Source: Volume 5 of *Wài Kē Fā Huī* 《外科發揮》 by Xuē Jǐ 薛己 *Míng* (明).

UF-9 Chái Hú Zhī Zǐ Sǎn 柴胡梔子散
Chái Hú and Zhī Zǐ Powder

治三焦及足少陽經風熱，耳內作癢生瘡，或出水疼痛，或胸乳間作痛，或寒熱往來 。

Treats wind-heat of the sān jiāo and the foot shǎoyàng channel with itching or sores inside the ears; or they discharge water with pain; or there is pain in the chest and breast region; or alternating chills and fever.

柴胡梔子（ 炒 ）牡丹皮（ 各一錢 ）茯苓川芎芍藥當歸牛蒡子
（ 炒，各七分 ）甘草（ 五分 ）

chái hú	柴胡		one qián	3.73 g
zhī zǐ	梔子	stir-fried	one qián	3.73 g
mǔ dān pí	牡丹皮		one qián	3.73 g
fú líng	茯苓		seven fēn	2.59 g
chuān xiōng	川芎		seven fēn	2.59 g
sháo yào	芍藥		seven fēn	2.59 g
dāng guī	當歸		seven fēn	2.59 g
niú bàng zǐ	牛蒡子	stir-fried	seven fēn	2.59 g
gān cǎo	甘草		five fēn	1.85 g

上水煎服。若太陽頭痛，加羌活。

Boil the above in water and take it. If it is a tàiyáng headache, add *qiāng huó*.

Source: Volume 4 of *Wài Kē Shū Yào* 《外科樞要》 by Xuē Jǐ 薛己 *Míng* (明).

UF-10 Fēng Liú Sǎn 風流散
Wind Flowing Powder

治損傷皮肉，血出不止，或破腦傷風，用藥填塞塗敷。

Treats injury to the skin and flesh with incessant bleeding; or brain-breaking tetanus.[95] Spread this medicine [over the wound] to completely fill it in.

血竭（二錢半，另研）番降真香節（四錢）燈心（一把）龍骨（二錢，另研）蘇木（少許，同降真另研）紅花（二錢，焙乾為末）當歸尾（三錢）乳香（半兩，同燈心研）沒藥（半兩，另研）新雞（一斤一隻，縛死不去毛雜，用醋煮半熟，砍碎，用好黃泥封固，谷殼文火煨乾，去骨末）桔梗（少許）

xuè jié	血竭	grind separately	2.5 qián	9.33 g
fān jiàng zhēn xiāng jié	番降真香節		four qián	14.92 g
dēng xīn	燈心			a handful
lóng gǔ	龍骨	grind separately	two qián	7.46 g
sū mù	蘇木	grind separately along with the jiàng zhēn		a small amount
hóng huā	紅花	stone-bake until dry, powder	two qián	7.46 g
dāng guī wěi	當歸尾		three qián	11.19 g
rǔ xiāng	乳香	grind with the dēng xīn	a half liǎng	18.65 g
mò yào	沒藥	grind separately	a half liǎng	18.65 g

---

95. *Pò nǎo shāng fēng* 破腦傷風 (brain-breaking tetanus): This is a condition with headache and then convulsions after an injury with broken skin or flesh.

xīn jī (a fresh chicken)	新雞	tie up and kill it without removing the feathers, boil in vinegar until half cooked, cut into pieces, seal it in mud from good yellow earth, roast until dried in a mild fire made from wheat chaff, remove the bones and powder them	one that weighs one jīn	596.8 g
jié gěng	桔梗			a small amount

上為細末，每用少許，乾摻瘡口上，如血流不止多摻之，候血藥將乾，又用清油調塗瘡口上。修合一料，以備急用。

Make the above into a fine powder. Each time, dry-sprinkle a little on the opening of the wound; if the bleeding does not stop, sprinkle a lot; wait until the blood and herbs are about to dry, then mix it with vegetable oil and smear it on the opening of the wound. Make a batch in advance to be prepared.

Source: The earliest recipe I can find for this is from 1556, twenty-seven years after *Zhèng Tǐ Lèi Yào* was published. This formula is probably similar to what Xuē Jǐ had in mind. It is from Volume 79 of *Gǔ Jīn Yī Tǒng Dà Quán* 《 古今醫統大全 》 by Xú Chūnfǔ 徐春甫 *Míng* (明).

Formulas that Xuē Jǐ said were Mistakenly Used

The following are mentioned as mistakenly used by by a patient. In some cases, Xuē Jǐ clearly disapproved of the formula as being too drastic. In other cases, the formula was simply used under the wrong circumstances. However, in this book, Xuē Jǐ never prescribed any of the following. A few come from books written or edited by Xuē Jǐ, so it is likely that he might have used those formulas in other situations.

UFx-1 Niú Huáng Qīng Xīn Wán 牛黃清心丸
Niú Huáng Heart-Clearing Decoction[96]

治諸風緩縱不隨，語言謇澀，心怔健忘，恍惚去來，頭目眩
冒，胸中煩鬱，痰涎壅塞，精神昏憒。又治心氣不足，神志
不定，驚恐怕怖，悲憂慘戚，虛煩少睡，喜怒無時；或發狂
顛，神情昏亂。

Treats all wind slackness with paralysis, difficulty speaking, palpitations, forgetfulness, abstraction that comes and goes, veiling dizziness of the head and eyes, vexation and constraint in the chest, phlegm-drool congestion, and muddled *jīng-shén*. It also treats insufficient heart qì, unstable *shén*-spirit and *zhì*-mind, fright, fear, sorrow, worry, heartache, and distress; deficiency vexation with little sleep, joy and anger at no particular time; or episodes of mania and withdrawal with muddled facial espression.

白芍藥麥門冬（去心）黃芩當歸（去苗）防風（去苗）白朮
（各一兩半）柴胡桔梗芎藭白茯苓（去皮）杏仁（去皮、
尖，麩炒黃，別研，各一兩二錢半）神曲（研）蒲黃（炒）
人參（去蘆，各二兩半）羚羊角末麝香（研）龍腦（研，各
一兩）肉桂（去粗皮）大豆黃卷（碎炒）阿膠（碎炒，各一
兩七錢半）白蘞乾薑（炮，各七錢半）牛黃（研，一兩二

---

96. This formula could not be used today without major modifications due to its use of endangered species, toxic ingredients, and expense.

173

錢 ）犀角末（ 二兩 ）雄黃（ 研飛，八錢 ）乾山藥（ 七兩 ）甘
草（ 銼，炒，五兩 ）金箔（ 一千二百箔，內四百箔爲衣 ）大
棗（ 一百枚，蒸熟去皮、核，研成膏 ）

bái sháo yào	白芍藥		1.5 liǎng	55.95 g
mài mén dōng	麥門冬	remove the core	1.5 liǎng	55.95 g
huáng qín	黃芩		1.5 liǎng	55.95 g
dāng guī	當歸	remove the sprouts	1.5 liǎng	55.95 g
fáng fēng	防風	remove the sprouts	1.5 liǎng	55.95 g
bái zhú	白朮		1.5 liǎng	55.95 g
chái hú	柴胡		1.25 liǎng	46.63 g
jié gěng	桔梗		1.25 liǎng	46.63 g
chuān xiōng	芎藭		1.25 liǎng	46.63 g
bái fú líng	白茯苓	remove the peel	1.25 liǎng	46.63 g
xìng rén	杏仁	remove the skin and tips, bran-fry until yellow, grind separately	1.25 liǎng	46.63 g
shén qū	神曲	grind	2.5 liǎng	93.25 g
pú huáng	蒲黃	stir-fry	2.5 liǎng	93.25 g
rén shēn	人參	remove the stem	2.5 liǎng	93.25 g
líng yáng jiǎo	羚羊角	powdered	one liǎng	37.3 g
shè xiāng	麝香	grind	one liǎng	37.3 g
lóng nǎo	龍腦	grind	one liǎng	37.3 g
ròu guì	肉桂	remove the coarse bark	1.75 liǎng	65.28 g
dà dòu huáng juàn	大豆黃卷	smash, stir-fry	1.75 liǎng	65.28 g
ē jiāo	阿膠	smash, stir-fry	1.75 liǎng	65.28 g
bái liǎn	白蘞		7.5 qián	28 g
gān jiāng	乾薑	blast-fry	7.5 qián	28 g
niú huáng	牛黃	grind	1.2 liǎng	44.8 g
xī jiǎo	犀角	powder	two liǎng	74.6 g
xióng huáng	雄黃	water grind	eight qián	29.84 g
gàn shān yào	乾山藥		seven liǎng	261.1 g
gān cǎo	甘草	cut, stir-fry	five liǎng	186.5 g
jīn bó	金箔	1,200 sheets; within this, 400 sheets as wrappers		
dà zǎo	大棗	steam until cooked, remove the skin and seeds, grind into a paste	100 pieces	

上除棗、杏仁、金箔、二角末及牛黃、麝香、雄黃、龍腦四
味外，為細末，入餘藥和勻，用煉蜜與棗膏為丸，每兩作一
十丸，用金箔為衣。每服一丸，溫水化下，食後服之。小兒
驚癇，即酌度多少，以竹葉湯溫溫化下。

Powder the above except the *zǎo*-dates, *xìng rén*, *jīn bó*, and two horns as well
as the four ingredients of *niú huáng, shè xiāng, xióng huáng, lóng nǎo*. Together,
make a fine powder, add in the rest of the powders and blend evenly. Make pills
with processed honey and the *zǎo*-date paste. Each *liǎng* of powder makes ten
pills. Use *jīn bó* as the outer wrapping. Each dose is one pill dissolved in warm
water and swallowed, taken after meals. For pediatric fright epilepsy, adjust the
amount; use a warm decoction of *zhú yè* to dissolve it and swallow it.

Source: Volume 1 of *Tài Píng Huì Mín Hé Jì Jú Fāng* 《太平惠民和劑局方》, the official
Sòng dynasty formulary.

UFx-2 Tòu Gǔ Dān 透骨丹
Bone-Piercing Elixir[97]

治諸風疼痛。

Treats all types of wind pain.

草烏（一兩，用塩和，炒焦）甘草（半兩）黑牽牛（一兩，
炒焦）

cǎo wū	草烏	blend with salt, stir-fry until burnt	one liǎng	37.3 g
gān cǎo	甘草		a half liǎng	18.65 g
hēi qiān niú	黑牽牛	stir-fry until burnt	one liǎng	37.3 g

右為末，加麝香一錢，和勻，酒糊為丸如梧桐子大。每服二
十丸，溫酒下，不拘時候。

Powder the above, add in one *qián* (3.73 grams) of *shè xiāng*, and blend evenly.
Make into pills the size of *wú tóng zǐ* (about 0.6-0.9 centimeters in diameter)

---

97. This formula cannot be used today because of its toxicity.

with wheat paste made using liquor. Each dose is twenty pills swallowed with warm liquor and taken at any time.

Source: Volume 116 of *Pǔ Jì Fāng*《普濟方》by Zhū Sù 朱橚 1406, *Míng* (明).

UFx-3 Fāng Mài Liú Qì Yǐn Zǐ 方脈流氣飲子
Qì-Flowing Drink for Miscellaneous Diseases

治惱怒胸膈脹滿；或肢體作痛；或結壅腫，血氣無虧者 。

Treats anger with distention and fullness of the chest and diaphragm, or painful body, or bindings, obstructions, and swellings without any lack of blood and qì.

紫蘇葉青皮苦梗半夏煨當歸芍藥烏藥茯苓川芎黃耆枳殼（ 去穰麩炒 ）防風（ 各半兩 ）甘草橘皮（ 各五分 ）大腹皮木香（ 各三分 ）

zǐ sū yè	紫蘇葉		a half liǎng	18.65 g
qīng pí	青皮		a half liǎng	18.65 g
kǔ gěng	苦梗		a half liǎng	18.65 g
bàn xià	半夏	roasted	a half liǎng	18.65 g
dāng guī	當歸		a half liǎng	18.65 g
sháo yào	芍藥		a half liǎng	18.65 g
wū yào	烏藥		a half liǎng	18.65 g
fú líng	茯苓		a half liǎng	18.65 g
chuān xiōng	川芎		a half liǎng	18.65 g
huáng qí	黃耆		a half liǎng	18.65 g
zhǐ qiào	枳殼	remove the pulp, stir-fry with wheat bran	a half liǎng	18.65 g
fang fēng	防風		a half liǎng	18.65 g
gān cǎo	甘草		five fēn	1.85 g
jú pí	橘皮		five fēn	1.85 g
dà fù pí	大腹皮		three fēn	1.11 g
mù xiāng	木香		three fēn	1.11 g

上薑棗水煎服 。

Boil the above in water with ginger and *zǎo*-dates and take it.

Source: Volume 1 of *Nǚ Kē Cuò Yào* 《 女科撮要 》 by Xuē Jǐ 薛己 *Míng* (明).

UFx-4 Bái Hǔ Tāng 白虎湯
White Tiger Decoction

治胃熱作渴，暑熱尤效；又治熱厥腹滿，身難轉側，面垢譫語，不時遺溺，手足厥冷，自汗，脈浮滑 。

Treats stomach heat with thirst. It is especially effective for summerheat; also treats hot *jué*-reversal with abdominal fullness, difficulty turning the body to the side, dirty complexion, raving speech, frequent incontinence of urine, *jué*-reversal cold of the hands and feet, spontaneous sweating, and floating slippery pulse.

知母，石膏（ 各二錢 ），粳米（ 半合 ）

zhī mǔ	知母	two qián	7.46 g
shí gāo	石膏	two qián	7.46 g
jīng mǐ	粳米	a half gě	29.84 g

上水煎服 。

Boil in water and take.

Source: Volume 7 of *Xiào Zhù Fù Rén Liáng Fāng* 《 校注婦人良方 》 by Xuē Jǐ 薛己 *Míng* (明).

Medicinals Index

A-Z Formulas Index

牛黃清心丸	*Niú Huáng Qīng Xīn Wán*	UFx-1	57, 173
七味白朮散	*Qī Wèi Bái Zhú Sǎn*	F-31	125
謙甫朱砂丸	*Qiān Fǔ Zhū Shā Wán*	F-68	155
羌活防風湯	*Qiāng Huó Fáng Fēng Tāng*	F-60	42, 65, 150
羌活湯	*Qiāng Huó Tāng*	F-63	42, 152
清暑益氣湯	*Qīng Shǔ Yì Qì Tāng*	UF-6	38, 167
清胃散	*Qīng Wèi Sǎn*	F-18	87, 114
清心蓮子飲	*Qīng Xīn Lián Zǐ Yǐn*	F-30	124
清燥湯	*Qīng Zào Tāng*	F-19	38, 77, 115
人參平肺散	*Rén Shēn Píng Fèi Sǎn*	F-27	98, 122
乳香定痛散	*Rǔ Xiāng Dìng Tòng Sǎn*	F-39	132
潤腸丸	*Rùn Cháng Wán*	F-13	39, 110
參附湯	*Shēn Fù Tāng*	F-17	30, 114
神效蔥熨法	*Shén Xiào Cōng Yùn Fǎ*	F-3	103
神效當歸膏	*Shén Xiào Dāng Guī Gāo*	F-41	98, 134
神效太乙膏	*Shén Xiào Tài Yǐ Gāo*	F-38	131
生脈散	*Shēng Mài Sǎn*	F-20	116
聖愈湯	*Shèng Yù Tāng*	F-15	33, 38, 73, 89, 112
十全大補湯	*Shí Quán Dà Bǔ Tāng*	F-16	11, 30, 32, 37–38, 46, 50, 56, 62, 68–69, 83, 88, 99, 113
十味參蘇飲	*Shí Wèi Shēn Sū Yǐn*	F-6	34, 105
四斤丸	*Sì Jīn Wán*	F-22	118
四君子湯	*Sì Jūn Zǐ Tāng*	F-1	11, 30, 33–35, 41, 59, 90, 99, 102, 128, 166
四生散	*Sì Shēng Sǎn*	F-24	120
四物湯	*Sì Wù Tāng*	F-8	11, 30, 35, 38–41, 46–47, 49, 52, 54, 62, 64, 67, 74–75, 77, 81, 87–88, 90, 92, 99–100, 107
四物參朮湯	*Sì Wù Shēn Zhú Tāng*	F-8	35
十全大補湯	*Shí Quán Dà Bǔ Tāng*	F-16	11, 30, 32, 37–38, 46, 50, 56, 62, 68–69, 83, 88, 99, 113
桃仁承氣湯	*Táo Rén Chéng Qì Tāng*	F-9	107

Sequential Formulas Index

F-1	四君子湯	Sì Jūn Zǐ Tāng	11, 30, 33–34, 41, 59, 90, 99, 102, 128, 166
F-2	小柴胡湯	Xiǎo Chái Hú Tāng	11, 28, 34, 41, 48, 51–52, 59, 61, 75, 77, 81, 85–86, 92, 103
F-3	神效蔥熨法	Shén Xiào [Cōng Yùn Fǎ]	78–79, 81, 87, 103
F-4	八珍湯	Bā Zhēn Tāng	11, 19, 30–32, 35, 37–38, 48, 58, 67, 73, 78, 81, 83, 85, 93, 98–99, 104
F-5	犀角地黃湯	Xī Jiǎo Dì Huáng Tāng	105, 143
F-6	十味參蘇飲	Shí Wèi Shēn Sū Yǐn	34, 105
F-6a	加味參蘇飲	Jiā Wèi Shēn Sū Yǐn	106
F-7	二味參蘇飲	Èr Wèi Shēn Sū Yǐn	34, 106
F-8	四物湯	Sì Wù Tāng	11, 30, 35, 38–41, 46–47, 49, 52, 54, 62, 64, 67, 74–75, 77, 81, 87–88, 90, 92, 99–100, 107
F-8a	加味四物湯	Jiā Wèi Sì Wù Tāng	30, 92, 107
F-9	桃仁承氣湯	Táo Rén Chéng Qì Tāng	107
F-9a	歸承湯	Guī Chéng Tāng	107
F-10	加味承氣湯	Jiā Wèi Chéng Qì Tāng	30, 108
F-11	獨參湯	Dú Shēn Tāng	33, 35, 39, 44, 46, 65, 67–68, 109
F-12	歸脾湯	Guī Pí Tāng	11, 46, 54, 67, 81, 109
F-12a	加味歸脾湯	Jiā Wèi Guī Pí Tāng	41, 110
F-13	潤腸丸	Rùn Cháng Wán	39, 110
F-14	當歸補血湯	Dāng Guī Bǔ Xuè Tāng	33, 46–47, 54, 111
F-15	聖愈湯	Shèng Yù Tāng	33, 38, 73, 89, 112
F-16	十全大補湯	Shí Quán Dà Bǔ Tāng	11, 30, 32, 37–38, 46, 50, 56, 62, 68–69, 83, 88, 99, 113
F-17	參附湯	Shēn Fù Tāng	30, 114
F-18	清胃散	Qīng Wèi Sǎn	87, 114
F-19	清燥湯	Qīng Zào Tāng	38, 77, 115

UF-3	二陳湯	*Èr Chén Tāng*	34, 41, 76–77, 166
UF-4	加味四君子湯	*Jiā Wèi Sì Jūn Zǐ Tāng*	35, 166
UF-5	調中益氣湯	*Tiáo Zhōng Yì Qì Tāng*	19, 38, 167
UF-6	清暑益氣湯	*Qīng Shǔ Yì Qì Tāng*	38, 167
UF-7	葛根湯	*Gé Gēn Tāng*	44, 168–169
UF-8	逍遙散	*Xiāo Yáo Sǎn*	101, 169
UF-9	柴胡梔子散	*Chái Hú Zhī Zǐ Sǎn*	140, 170
UF-10	風流散	*Fēng Liú Sǎn*	142, 171
UFx-1	牛黃清心丸	*Niú Huáng Qīng Xīn Wán*	57, 173
UFx-2	透骨丹	*Tòu Gǔ Dān*	20, 76, 175
UFx-3	流氣飲	*Liú Qì Yǐn*	82–83, 176
UFx-3	方脈流氣飲子	*Fāng Mài Liú Qì Yǐn Zǐ*	176
UFx-4	白虎湯	*Bái Hǔ Tāng*	47, 111, 177

Diagnosis & Corresponding Formula in Vol. 1

abundance of phlegm-drool congesting	F-65	*Dà Xiōng Huáng Tāng*	43
abundance of phlegm-fire	UF-3	*Èr Chén Tāng*	34
already developed pus			31
anger injuring the liver	F-2	*Xiǎo Chái Hú Tāng*	52
binding constraint of spleen qì	F-12a	*Jiā Wèi Guī Pí Tāng*	41
blood and qì are injured	F-8	*Sì Wù Tāng*	30
blood deficiency leading to liver distention	F-8	*Sì Wù Tāng*	52
blood deficiency with agitation	F-14	*Dāng Guī Bǔ Xuè Tāng*	46–47
blood desertion with vexation and agitation	F-11	*Dú Shēn Tāng*	45
blood heat to disorder the channels and move recklessly	UF-1	*Jiā Wèi Xiāo Yáo Sǎn*	35
blood stagnation of the liver channel	F-8	*Sì Wù Tāng*	41
blood stasis is developing into pus	F-4	*Bā Zhēn Tāng*	32
blood stasis is not completely removed	F-8a	*Jiā Wèi Sì Wù Tāng*	30
blood stasis is present internally	F-10	*Jiā Wèi Chéng Qì Tāng*	30
blood stasis on the inside	F-41	*Dāng Guī Gāo*	50
blood stasis that collects and stagnates	F-44	*Dāng Guī Dǎo Zhì Sǎn*	28
blood taking advantage of qì deficiency in the lungs	F-7	*Èr Wèi Shēn Sū Yǐn*	34
collapse of blood	F-15	*Shèng Yù Tāng*	33, 74–75
collapse of *jīnyè*-fluids			43
conquered spleen and stomach qì			31
constrained fire of the liver channel	F-2	*Xiǎo Chái Hú Tāng*	58–59
deficiency heat of the kidney channel	F-29	*Dì Huáng Wán*	35
deficiency of both qì and blood	F-16	*Shí Quán Dà Bǔ Tāng*	43, 47, 50, 90, 96
deficiency of both qì and blood with evil fire blazing vigorously	F-8	*Sì Wù Tāng*	47
deficiency of qì and blood in the liver and gallbladder			53
deficiency of yīn and blood in the lower body			75
deficiency condition of both the physical body and qì	F-34	*Liù Jūn Zǐ Tāng*	61

192

qì counterflow with blood amassing in the lungs	F-6	*Shí Wèi Shēn Sū Yǐn*	34
soft tetany	F-67	*Bái Zhú Tāng*	44
spleen and kidneys are extremely deficient and cold	F-17	*Shēn Fù Tāng*	30
spleen and kidneys are injured	F-34	*Liù Jūn Zǐ Tāng*	30
spleen and lung qì are deficient	F-23	*Bǔ Zhōng Yì Qì Tāng*	38
spleen and lung qì are stagnant	UF-3	*Èr Chén Tāng*	41
spleen and lung qì deficiency	F-4	*Bā Zhēn Tāng*	31
spleen and stomach qì are deficient	F-34	*Liù Jūn Zǐ Tāng*	38
spleen and stomach qì deficiency	F-23	*Bǔ Zhōng Yì Qì Tāng*	31
spleen and stomach qì desertion			31
spleen qì is deficient	F-34	*Liù Jūn Zǐ Tāng*	38
stagnation of *yíng* and *wèi* qì	F-37	*Fù Yuán Tōng Qì Sǎn*	31
static blood streaming sores	F-2	*Xiǎo Chái Hú Tāng*	48
stomach deficiency with insufficient *jīnyè*-fluids	F-23	*Bǔ Zhōng Yì Qì Tāng*	35
stomach heat injuring jīnyè-fluids	F-25	*Zhú Yè Huáng Qí Tāng*	35
stomach fire blazing vigorously			35
stomach qì deficiency	F-23	*Bǔ Zhōng Yì Qì Tāng*	31, 34
stomach qì is injured	F-34	*Liù Jūn Zǐ Tāng*	30
tetany wind disease			43
unrooted deficiency fire			33
yáng qì is deficient and cold	F-17	*Shēn Fù Tāng*	30
yáng qì is injured	F-16	*Shí Quán Dà Bǔ Tāng*	30
yīn and blood are deficient	F-8	*Sì Wù Tāng*	38
yīn and blood are injured	F-8	*Sì Wù Tāng*	30
yīn and blood have received injury	F-8	*Sì Wù Tāng*	49
yīn deficiency	F-14	*Dāng Guī Bǔ Xuè Tāng*	33
yīn exuberance with agitation	F-1	*Sì Jūn Zǐ Tāng*	33

194

General Index

201

The Chinese Medicine Database

www.cm-db.com

The Chinese Medicine Database has been organized around one central principle -- translation of Classical Asian texts, and dissemination of that information.

There are thousands of Asian medicine texts that have never been translated. We have compiled a small list on our website of the ones that we have found, but we believe that there are tens of thousands of documents that span from the *Hàn* Dynasty to pre-Republican times. Most of these documents will never be read by people in the West, simply because of lack of translation.

We have created a vehicle, that allows interested practitioners, students, institutions, and scholars to help support and fund the translation of these documents, and then mine and synthesize the data that is gained from these texts.

The Database contains:

Monographs on:
690 Single Herbs
1510 Formulas
Mayway's Patents
ITM's Formulations
Golden Flowers Formulations
Classical Pearls Formulations by Heiner Fruehauf
OBGYN Modifications to Formulas
Single Points: the 361 Regular Points
Time Line of the History of Chinese Medicine

Beer Hall Lecture Series:
Watch videos from our monthly Beer Hall lecture series with guest speakers such as: Arnaud Versluys, Subhuti Dharmananda, Jason Robertson, Craig Mitchell, Michael Max, Lorraine Wilcox, and Ed Neal.

CEU/ PDA/ Livestreaming Lectures:
We now have a stand alone video system which allows people to watch lectures without being a subscriber. These lectures feature top quality lecturers speaking on classical Chinese medicine and medicinals. This can be found at: http://cm-db.com/xstreaming.php

Play STORT:

Play our free online game STORT where you can learn Chinese while having a bit of fun (www.cm-db.com/stort).

A Chinese-English dictionary:

Containing over 105,000 terms, including the Eastland and the WHO term sets.

Our Translation Tools:

A pop-up translation system using the terminology in our books, as well as our Chinese-English dictionary system. This allows the user to translate their own documents out of Chinese.

Translations:

Shāng Hán Lái Sū Jí	傷寒來蘇集	Renewal of Treatise on Cold Damage
Qí Jīng Bā Mài Kǎo	奇經八脈考	Explanation of the Eight Vessels of the Marvellous Meridians
Shāng Hán Míng Lǐ Lùn	傷寒明理論	Treatise on Enlightening the Principles of Cold Damage
Wú Jū Tōng Yī Àn	吴鞠通医案	Case Studies of Wú Jūtōng
The Nàn Jīng	難經	The Classic of Difficulties
The Zàng Fǔ Biāo Běn Hán Rè Xū Shí Yòng Yào Shì	臟腑標本寒熱虚實用藥式	Viscera and Bowels, Tip and Root, Cold and Heat, Vacuity and Repletion Model for Using Medicinals
Wēn Rè Lún	温熱論	Treatise on Warm Heat Disease
Shāng Hán Shé Jiàn	傷寒舌鑒	Tongue Mirror of Cold Damage
Xǔ Shì Yī Àn	許氏醫案	Case Histories of Master Xǔ
Fǔ Xíng Jué Zāng Fǔ Yòng Yào Fǎ Yào	輔行決臟腑用藥法要	Secret Instructions for Assisting the Body: Essential Methods for the Application of Drugs to the Viscera & Bowels
Biāo Yōu Fù	標幽賦	Indicating the Obscure
Liú Juān Zǐ Guǐ Yí Fāng	劉涓子鬼遺方	Liu Juanzi's Formulas Inherited from Ghosts
Shèn Jí Chú Yán	慎疾芻言	Precautions in Illness: My Humble Thoughts
Yào Zhèng Jì Yí	藥症忌宜	Medicinals & Patterns Contraindications & Appropriate [Choices]
Fù Kē Wèn Dá	婦科問答	Questions and Answers in Gynecology
Nèi Jīng Zhī Yào	內經知要	Essential Knowledge from the Nèijīng

| Běn Cǎo Bèi Yào | 本草備要 | The Essential Completion of Traditional Materia Medica |
| Bǎi Zhèng Fù (Jù Yīng) | 百症賦《聚英》 | Ode of the Hundred Diseases from The Great Compendium of Acupuncture-Moxibustion |

Benefits:

Subscribers to the Database receive a 10% discount on our published books when they are in pre-release.

Published Books:

2008 Bèi Jí Qiān Jīn Yào Fāng 備急千金要方:
Essential Prescriptions Worth a Thousand Gold Pieces For Emergencies. vol. 2-4
by Sūn Sīmiǎo 孫思邈
Translated by Sabine Wilms.
ISBN 978-0-9799552-0-4
Permanently Out of Print

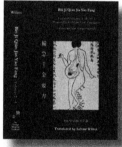

2010 Zhēn Jiǔ Dà Chéng 針灸大成:
The Great Compendium of Acupuncture & Moxibustion vol. I
by Yáng Jìzhōu 楊繼洲
Translated by Sabine Wilms.
ISBN 978-0-9799552-2-8

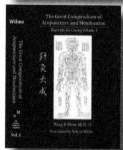

2010 Zhēn Jiǔ Dà Chéng 針灸大成:
The Great Compendium of Acupuncture & Moxibustion vol. V
by Yáng Jìzhōu 楊繼洲
Translated by Lorraine Wilcox.
ISBN 978-0-9799552-4-2

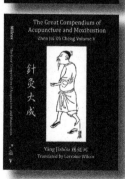

2010 Jīn Guì Fāng Gē Kuò 金匱方歌括:
Formulas from the Golden Cabinet with Songs vol. I - III
by Chén Xiūyuán 陳修園
Translated by Sabine Wilms.
ISBN 978-0-9799552-5-9

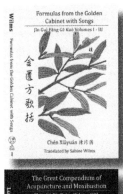

2011 Zhēn Jiǔ Dà Chéng 針灸大成:
The Great Compendium of Acupuncture & Moxibustion
vol. VIII
by Yáng Jìzhōu 楊繼洲
Translated by Yue Lu.
ISBN 978-0-9799552-7-3

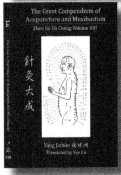

2011 Zhēn Jiǔ Dà Chéng 針灸大成:
The Great Compendium of Acupuncture & Moxibustion
vol. IX
by Yáng Jìzhōu 楊繼洲
Translated by Lorraine Wilcox.
ISBN 978-0-9799552-6-6

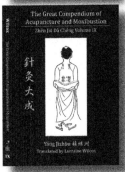

2012 Raising the Dead and Returning Life: Emergency
Medicine of the Qīng Dynasty
by Bào Xiāng'áo 鮑相璈
Translated by Lorraine Wilcox.
ISBN 978-0-9799552-3-5

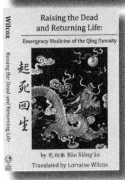

2014 Zhēn Jiǔ Zī Shēng Jīng 針灸資生經:
The Classic of Supporting Life with Acupuncture and
Moxibustion Vol. I-III
by Wáng Zhízhōng 王執中
Translated by Yue Lu.
ISBN 978-0-9799552-1-1

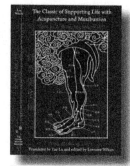

2014 Jīn Guì Fāng Gē Kuò 金匱方歌括:
Formulas from the Golden Cabinet with Songs
vol. IV - VI
by Chén Xiūyuán 陳修園
Translated by Eran Even.
ISBN 978-0-9799552-8-0

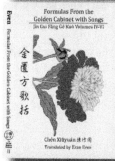

2015 Zhēn Jiǔ Zī Shēng Jīng 針灸資生經:
The Classic of Supporting Life with Acupuncture and Moxi-
bustion Vol. IV-VII
by Wáng Zhízhōng 王執中
Translated by Yue Lu.
ISBN 978-0-9799552-9-7

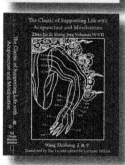

2015 Nǚ Yī Zá Yán 女醫雜言:
Miscellaneous Records of a Female Doctor
by Tán Yǔnxián 談允賢
Translated by Lorraine Wilcox.
ISBN 978-0-9906029-0-3

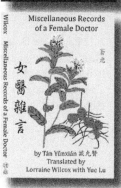

2016 Nǔ Kē Cuō Yào 女科撮要:
Outline of Female Medicine
by Xuē Jǐ 薛己
Translated by Lorraine Wilcox.
ISBN 978-0-9906029-1-0

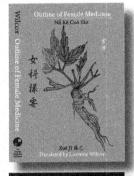

2016 Shén Nóng Běn Cǎo Jīng Dú 神農本草經讀:
Reading of the Divine Farmer's Classic of Materia Medica
by Chén Xiūyuán 陳修園
Translated by Corinna Theisinger.
ISBN 978-0-9906029-2-7

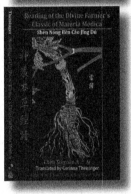

CPSIA information can be obtained
at www.ICGtesting.com
Printed in the USA
BVOW09s1225071117
499763BV00021B/1160/P